D1505163

More short stories available
from Macmillan Collector's Library

SLEEPILY EVER AFTER

Bedtime Stories for Grown Ups

Edited and introduced by
ZACHARY SEAGER

MACMILLAN COLLECTOR'S LIBRARY

This collection first published 2021 by Macmillan Collector's Library
an imprint of Pan Macmillan
The Smithson, 6 Briset Street, London EC1M 5NR
EU representative: Macmillan Publishers Ireland Limited, 1st Floor,
The Liffey Trust Centre, 117–126 Sheriff Street Upper,
Dublin 1, DO1 YC43
Associated companies throughout the world
www.panmacmillan.com

ISBN 978-1-5290-7077-4

Selection and arrangement copyright © Macmillan Publishers International Limited 2021

Introduction copyright © Zachary Seager 2021

3 5 7 9 8 6 4

A CIP catalogue record for this book is available from the British Library.

Cover and endpaper design: Mel Four, Pan Macmillan Art Department
Typeset in Plantin by Jouve (UK), Milton Keynes
Printed and bound in China by Imago

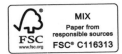

MIX
Paper from
responsible sources
FSC® C116313

Visit **www.panmacmillan.com** to read more
about all our books and to buy them.

Contents

Introduction

The world can be a frightening place. You hear it on the news every day. You see it on your phone screen late at night, in those exasperating hours when, with a heavy sigh, sleep escapes your yearning grasp. Looking for peace, calm, and hope, you search for a good book to help you drift off.

But most of the books you find are depressing, distressing, or just plain dull. And rightly so, it is argued. Happy endings, uplifting fictions, and tales with a clear moral resolution are for children, we are told. Life is not like that. Growing up means accepting this fact, as well as its corollary: literature depicts life as it is, in all its depressing, distressing, dull majesty.

Even so, you catch yourself longing for an earlier time, when you could enjoy without a cynical scoff a story about Snow White or Sleeping Beauty. *If only I could see the world with innocent eyes again!* you think. *If only I could thrill once more to Peter Pan's adventures and dreamily contemplate a love like Cinderella's.* But those tales are too simple, you believe; and in any case, you are too mature, too sophisticated for them now. Back to the depressing, distressing, and dull, then; back to troubled sleep and the frightening world.

But just as the world is far less frightening than the news would have you believe, this story of literature is misleading too. Literature, like life, can be uplifting without being simplistic; illuminating without being depressing; and morally good without being deathly dull.

In fact, although there are clear historical reasons why journeys into the literary heart of darkness have taken artistic precedence – most notably the triumph of literary modernism's values in universities, prize-giving organizations, and other taste-making institutions – there is also a technical reason why gloomy books predominate: it is exceptionally difficult to write a successful, positive story—especially one that is resolutely aimed at adults. Proving engaging and joyful, and at the same time true to life; avoiding sentimentality and fairy-tale wish fulfilment while remaining credible; these are some of the toughest tests a writer can face.

This is where *Sleepily Ever After: Bedtime Stories for Grown Ups* comes in. Collecting together classic stories by great writers as well as delightful tales by lesser-known authors, the works in this anthology are by turns touching, upbeat, humorous, and inspiring. They consistently rise to the literary challenge posed by the pleasing, positive story; and they are always and above all entertaining.

From Japanese folktales to Virginia Woolf, from Louisa May Alcott to F. Scott Fitzgerald, the stories in this volume will make you smile and help you relax, allowing you to gently fall asleep with a contented grin and a peaceful mind.

SLEEPILY EVER AFTER

OSCAR WILDE

The Model Millionaire

Unless one is wealthy there is no use in being a charming fellow. Romance is the privilege of the rich, not the profession of the unemployed. The poor should be practical and prosaic. It is better to have a permanent income than to be fascinating. These are the great truths of modern life which Hughie Erskine never realised. Poor Hughie! Intellectually, we must admit, he was not of much importance. He never said a brilliant or even an ill-natured thing in his life. But then he was wonderfully good-looking, with his crisp brown hair, his clear-cut profile, and his grey eyes. He was as popular with men as he was with women and he had every accomplishment except that of making money. His father had bequeathed him his cavalry sword and a *History of the Peninsular War* in fifteen volumes. Hughie hung the first over his looking-glass, put the second on a shelf between *Ruff's Guide* and *Bailey's Magazine*, and lived on two hundred a year that an old aunt allowed him. He had tried everything. He had gone on the Stock Exchange for six months; but what was a butterfly to do among bulls and bears? He had been a tea-merchant for a little longer, but had soon tired of pekoe and souchong. Then he had tried selling dry sherry. That did not answer; the sherry was a little too dry. Ultimately he became nothing, a delightful, ineffectual young man with a perfect profile and no profession.

To make matters worse, he was in love. The girl he

loved was Laura Merton, the daughter of a retired Colonel who had lost his temper and his digestion in India, and had never found either of them again. Laura adored him, and he was ready to kiss her shoe-strings. They were the handsomest couple in London, and had not a penny-piece between them. The Colonel was very fond of Hughie, but would not hear of any engagement.

"Come to me, my boy, when you have got ten thousand pounds of your own, and we will see about it," he used to say; and Hughie looked very glum in those days, and had to go to Laura for consolation.

One morning, as he was on his way to Holland Park, where the Mertons lived, he dropped in to see a great friend of his, Alan Trevor. Trevor was a painter. Indeed, few people escape that nowadays. But he was also an artist, and artists are rather rare. Personally he was a strange rough fellow, with a freckled face and a red ragged beard. However, when he took up the brush he was a real master, and his pictures were eagerly sought after. He had been very much attracted by Hughie at first, it must be acknowledged, entirely on account of his personal charm. "The only people a painter should know," he used to say, "are people who are *bête* and beautiful, people who are an artistic pleasure to look at and an intellectual repose to talk to. Men who are dandies and women who are darlings rule the world, at least they should do so." However, after he got to know Hughie better, he liked him quite as much for his bright, buoyant spirits and his generous, reckless nature, and had given him the permanent *entrée* to his studio.

When Hughie came in he found Trevor putting the finishing touches to a wonderful life-size picture of a beggar-man. The beggar himself was standing on a raised platform in a corner of the studio. He was a wizened old man, with a face like wrinkled parchment, and a most piteous expression. Over his shoulders was flung a coarse brown cloak, all tears and tatters; his thick boots were patched and cobbled, and with one hand he leant on a rough stick, while with the other he held out his battered hat for alms.

"What an amazing model!" whispered Hughie, as he shook hands with his friend.

"An amazing model?" shouted Trevor at the top of his voice; "I should think so! Such beggars as he are not to be met with every day. A *trouvaille, mon cher*; a living Velasquez! My stars! what an etching Rembrandt would have made of him!"

"Poor old chap!" said Hughie, "how miserable he looks! But I suppose, to you painters, his face is his fortune?"

"Certainly," replied Trevor, "you don't want a beggar to look happy, do you?"

"How much does a model get for sitting?" asked Hughie, as he found himself a comfortable seat on a divan.

"A shilling an hour."

"And how much do you get for your picture, Alan?"

"Oh, for this I get two thousand!"

"Pounds?"

"Guineas. Painters, poets, and physicians always get guineas."

"Well, I think the model should have a percentage," cried Hughie, laughing; "they work quite as hard as you do."

"Nonsense, nonsense! Why, look at the trouble of laying on the paint alone, and standing all day long at one's easel! It's all very well, Hughie, for you to talk, but I assure you that there are moments when Art

3

almost attains to the dignity of manual labour. But you mustn't chatter; I'm very busy. Smoke a cigarette, and keep quiet."

After some time the servant came in, and told Trevor that the framemaker wanted to speak to him.

"Don't run away, Hughie," he said, as he went out, "I will be back in a moment."

The old beggar-man took advantage of Trevor's absence to rest for a moment on a wooden bench that was behind him. He looked so forlorn and wretched that Hughie could not help pitying him, and felt in his pockets to see what money he had. All he could find was a sovereign and some coppers. "Poor old fellow," he thought to himself, "he wants it more than I do, but it means no hansoms for a fortnight"; and he walked across the studio and slipped the sovereign into the beggar's hand.

The old man started, and a faint smile flitted across his withered lips. "Thank you, sir," he said, "thank you."

Then Trevor arrived, and Hughie took his leave, blushing a little at what he had done. He spent the day with Laura, got a charming scolding for his extravagance, and had to walk home.

That night he strolled into the Palette Club about eleven o'clock, and found Trevor sitting by himself in the smoking-room drinking hock and seltzer.

"Well, Alan, did you get the picture finished all right?" he said, as he lit his cigarette.

"Finished and framed, my boy!" answered Trevor; "and, by the bye, you have made a conquest. That old model you saw is quite devoted to you. I had to tell him all about you—who you are, where you live, what your income is, what prospects you have—"

"My dear Alan," cried Hughie, "I shall probably find

him waiting for me when I go home. But of course you are only joking. Poor old wretch! I wish I could do something for him. I think it is dreadful that anyone should be so miserable. I have got heaps of old clothes at home—do you think he would care for any of them? Why, his rags were falling to bits."

"But he looks splendid in them," said Trevor. "I wouldn't paint him in a frock coat for anything. What you call rags I call romance. What seems poverty to you is picturesqueness to me. However, I'll tell him of your offer."

"Alan," said Hughie seriously, "you painters are a heartless lot."

"An artist's heart is his head," replied Trevor; "and besides, our business is to realise the world as we see it, not to reform it as we know it. *À chacun son métier.* And now tell me how Laura is. The old model was quite interested in her."

"You don't mean to say you talked to him about her?" said Hughie.

"Certainly I did. He knows all about the relentless colonel, the lovely Laura, and the £10,000."

"You told that old beggar all my private affairs?" cried Hughie, looking very red and angry.

"My dear boy," said Trevor, smiling, "that old beggar, as you call him, is one of the richest men in Europe. He could buy all London to-morrow without overdrawing his account. He has a house in every capital, dines off gold plate, and can prevent Russia going to war when he chooses."

"What on earth do you mean?" exclaimed Hughie.

"What I say," said Trevor. "The old man you saw to-day in the studio was Baron Hausberg. He is a great friend of mine, buys all my pictures and that sort of thing, and gave me a commission a month ago to paint him as a beggar. *Que voulez-vous? La fantaisie d'un millionnaire!* And I must say he made a magnificent figure in his rags, or perhaps I should say in my rags; they are an old suit I got in Spain."

"Baron Hausberg!" cried Hughie. "Good heavens! I gave him a sovereign!" and he sank into an armchair the picture of dismay.

"Gave him a sovereign!" shouted Trevor, and he burst into a roar of laughter. "My dear boy, you'll never see it again. *Son affaire c'est l'argent des autres.*"

"I think you might have told me, Alan," said Hughie sulkily, "and not have let me make such a fool of myself."

"Well, to begin with, Hughie," said Trevor, "it never entered my mind that you went about distributing alms in that reckless way. I can understand your kissing a pretty model, but your giving a sovereign to an ugly one—by Jove, no! Besides, the fact is that I really was not at home to-day to anyone; and when you came in I didn't know whether Hausberg would like his name mentioned. You know he wasn't in full dress."

"What a duffer he must think me!" said Hughie.

"Not at all. He was in the highest spirits after you left; kept chuckling to himself and rubbing his old wrinkled hands together. I couldn't make out why he was so interested to know all about you; but I see it all now. He'll invest your sovereign for you, Hughie, pay you the interest every six months, and have a capital story to tell after dinner."

"I am an unlucky devil," growled Hughie. "The best thing I can do is to go to bed; and, my dear Alan, you mustn't tell anyone. I shouldn't dare show my face in the Row."

"Nonsense! It reflects the highest credit on your

philanthropic spirit, Hughie. And don't run away. Have another cigarette, and you can talk about Laura as much as you like."

However, Hughie wouldn't stop, but walked home, feeling very unhappy, and leaving Alan Trevor in fits of laughter.

The next morning, as he was at breakfast, the servant brought him up a card on which was written, "Monsieur Gustave Naudin, *de la part de* M. le Baron Hausberg."

"I suppose he has come for an apology," said Hughie to himself; and he told the servant to show the visitor up.

An old gentleman with gold spectacles and grey hair came into the room, and said, in a slight French accent, "Have I the honour of addressing Monsieur Erskine?"

Hughie bowed.

"I have come from Baron Hausberg," he continued. "The Baron—"

"I beg, sir, that you will offer him my sincerest apologies," stammered Hughie.

"The Baron," said the old gentleman with a smile, "has commissioned me to bring you this letter"; and he extended a sealed envelope.

On the outside was written, "A wedding present to Hugh Erskine and Laura Merton, from an old beggar," and inside was a cheque for £10,000.

When they were married Alan Trevor was the best man, and the Baron made a speech at the wedding breakfast.

"Millionaire models," remarked Alan, "are rare enough; but, by Jove, model millionaires are rarer still!"

KATE CHOPIN

A Pair of Silk Stockings

Little Mrs. Sommers one day found herself the unexpected possessor of fifteen dollars. It seemed to her a very large amount of money, and the way in which it stuffed and bulged her worn old *porte-monnaie* gave her a feeling of importance such as she had not enjoyed for years.

The question of investment was one that occupied her greatly. For a day or two she walked about apparently in a dreamy state, but really absorbed in speculation and calculation. She did not wish to act hastily, to do anything she might afterward regret. But it was during the still hours of the night when she lay awake revolving plans in her mind that she seemed to see her way clearly toward a proper and judicious use of the money.

A dollar or two should be added to the price usually paid for Janie's shoes, which would ensure their lasting an appreciable time longer than they usually did. She would buy so and so many yards of percale for new shirt waists for the boys and Janie and Mag. She had intended to make the old ones do by skilful patching. Mag should have another gown. She had seen some beautiful patterns, veritable bargains in the shop windows. And still there would be left enough for new stockings—two pairs apiece—and what darning that would save for a while! She would get caps for the boys and sailor-hats for the girls. The vision of her little

9

brood looking fresh and dainty and new for once in their lives excited her and made her restless and wakeful with anticipation.

The neighbours sometimes talked of certain "better days" that little Mrs. Sommers had known before she had ever thought of being Mrs. Sommers. She herself indulged in no such morbid retrospection. She had no time—no second of time to devote to the past. The needs of the present absorbed her every faculty. A vision of the future like some dim, gaunt monster sometimes appalled her, but luckily to-morrow never comes.

Mrs. Sommers was one who knew the value of bargains; who could stand for hours making her way inch by inch toward the desired object that was selling below cost. She could elbow her way if need be; she had learned to clutch a piece of goods and hold it and stick to it with persistence and determination till her turn came to be served, no matter when it came.

But that day she was a little faint and tired. She had swallowed a light luncheon—no! when she came to think of it, between getting the children fed and the place righted, and preparing herself for the shopping bout, she had actually forgotten to eat any luncheon at all!

She sat herself upon a revolving stool before a counter that was comparatively deserted, trying to gather strength and courage to charge through an eager multitude that was besieging breastworks of shirting and figured lawn. An all-gone limp feeling had come over her and she rested her hand aimlessly upon the counter. She wore no gloves. By degrees she grew aware that her hand had encountered something very soothing, very pleasant to touch. She looked down to see that her hand lay upon a pile of silk stockings. A placard near by announced that they had been reduced in price from two dollars and fifty cents to one dollar and ninety-eight cents; and a young girl who stood behind the counter asked her if she wished to examine their line of silk hosiery. She smiled, just as if she had been asked to inspect a tiara of diamonds with the ultimate view of purchasing it. But she went on feeling the soft, sheeny luxurious things—with both hands now, holding them up to see them glisten, and to feel them glide serpent-like through her fingers.

Two hectic blotches came suddenly into her pale cheeks. She looked up at the girl.

"Do you think there are any eights-and-a-half among these?"

There were any number of eights-and-a-half. In fact, there were more of that size than any other. Here was a light-blue pair; there were some lavender, some all black and various shades of tan and grey. Mrs. Sommers selected a black pair and looked at them very long and closely. She pretended to be examining their texture, which the clerk assured her was excellent.

"A dollar and ninety-eight cents," she mused aloud. "Well, I'll take this pair." She handed the girl a five-dollar bill and waited for her change and for her parcel. What a very small parcel it was! It seemed lost in the depths of her shabby old shopping-bag.

Mrs. Sommers after that did not move in the direction of the bargain counter. She took the elevator, which carried her to an upper floor into the region of the ladies' waiting-rooms. Here, in a retired corner, she exchanged her cotton stockings for the new silk ones which she had just bought. She was not going through any acute mental process or reasoning with herself, nor was she striving to explain to her satisfaction the motive of her action. She was not thinking at all. She seemed for the time to be taking a rest from that laborious and fatiguing function and to have abandoned herself to some mechanical impulse that directed her actions and freed her of responsibility.

How good was the touch of the raw silk to her flesh! She felt like lying back in the cushioned chair and revelling for a while in the luxury of it. She did for a little while. Then she replaced her shoes, rolled the cotton stockings together and thrust them into her bag. After doing this she crossed straight over to the shoe department and took her seat to be fitted.

She was fastidious. The clerk could not make her out; he could not reconcile her shoes with her stockings, and she was not too easily pleased. She held back her skirts and turned her feet one way and her head another way as she glanced down at the polished, pointed-tipped boots. Her foot and ankle looked very pretty. She could not realize that they belonged to her and were a part of herself. She wanted an excellent and stylish fit, she told the young fellow who served her, and she did not mind the difference of a dollar or two more in the price so long as she got what she desired.

It was a long time since Mrs. Sommers had been fitted with gloves. On rare occasions when she had bought a pair they were always "bargains," so cheap that it would have been preposterous and unreasonable to have expected them to be fitted to the hand.

Now she rested her elbow on the cushion of the glove counter, and a pretty, pleasant young creature, delicate and deft of touch, drew a long-wristed "kid" over Mrs. Sommers's hand. She smoothed it down over the wrist and buttoned it neatly, and both lost themselves for a second or two in admiring contemplation of the little symmetrical gloved hand. But there were other places where money might be spent.

There were books and magazines piled up in the window of a stall a few paces down the street. Mrs. Sommers bought two high-priced magazines such as she had been accustomed to read in the days when she had been accustomed to other pleasant things. She carried them without wrapping. As well as she could she lifted her skirts at the crossings. Her stockings and boots and well-fitting gloves had worked marvels in her bearing— had given her a feeling of assurance, a sense of belonging to the well-dressed multitude.

She was very hungry. Another time she would have stilled the cravings for food until reaching her own home, where she would have brewed herself a cup of tea and taken a snack of anything that was available. But the impulse that was guiding her would not suffer her to entertain any such thought.

There was a restaurant at the corner. She had never entered its doors; from the outside she had sometimes caught glimpses of spotless damask and shining crystal, and soft-stepping waiters serving people of fashion.

When she entered her appearance created no surprise, no consternation, as she had half feared it might. She seated herself at a small table alone, and an attentive waiter at once approached to take her order. She did not want a profusion; she craved a nice and tasty bite—a half dozen blue-points, a plump chop with cress, a something sweet—a *crème-frappée*, for instance; a glass of Rhine wine, and after all a small cup of black coffee.

While waiting to be served she removed her gloves very leisurely and laid them beside her. Then she picked up a magazine and glanced through it, cutting the pages with a blunt edge of her knife. It was all very agreeable.

The damask was even more spotless than it had seemed through the window, and the crystal more sparkling. There were quiet ladies and gentlemen, who did not notice her, lunching at the small tables like her own. A soft, pleasing strain of music could be heard, and a gentle breeze was blowing through the window. She tasted a bite, and she read a word or two, and she sipped the amber wine and wiggled her toes in the silk stockings. The price of it made no difference. She counted the money out to the waiter and left an extra coin on his tray, whereupon he bowed before her as before a princess of royal blood.

There was still money in her purse, and her next temptation presented itself in the shape of a matinee poster.

It was a little later when she entered the theatre, the play had begun and the house seemed to her to be packed. But there were vacant seats here and there, and into one of them she was ushered, between brilliantly dressed women who had gone there to kill time and eat candy and display their gaudy attire. There were many others who were there solely for the play and acting. It is safe to say there was no one present who bore quite the attitude which Mrs. Sommers did to her surroundings. She gathered in the whole—stage and players and people in one wide impression, and absorbed it and enjoyed it. She laughed at the comedy and wept—she and the gaudy woman next to her wept over the tragedy. And they talked a little together over it. And the gaudy woman wiped her eyes and sniffled on a tiny square of filmy, perfumed lace and passed little Mrs. Sommers her box of candy.

The play was over, the music ceased, the crowd filed out. It was like a dream ended. People scattered in all directions. Mrs. Sommers went to the corner and waited for the cable car.

A man with keen eyes, who sat opposite to her, seemed to like the study of her small, pale face. It puzzled him to decipher what he saw there. In truth, he saw nothing—unless he were wizard enough to detect a poignant wish, a powerful longing that the cable car would never stop anywhere, but go on and on with her forever.

O. HENRY

The Ransom of Red Chief

It looked like a good thing: but wait till I tell you. We were down South, in Alabama—Bill Driscoll and myself—when this kidnapping idea struck us. It was, as Bill afterward expressed it, "during a moment of temporary mental apparition"; but we didn't find that out till later.

There was a town down there, as flat as a flannel-cake, and called Summit, of course. It contained inhabitants of as undeleterious and self-satisfied a class of peasantry as ever clustered around a Maypole.

Bill and me had a joint capital of about six hundred dollars, and we needed just two thousand dollars more to pull off a fraudulent town-lot scheme in Western Illinois with. We talked it over on the front steps of the hotel. Philoprogenitiveness, says we, is strong in semi-rural communities; therefore and for other reasons, a kidnapping project ought to do better there than in the radius of newspapers that send reporters out in plain clothes to stir up talk about such things. We knew that Summit couldn't get after us with anything stronger than constables and maybe some lackadaisical blood-hounds and a diatribe or two in the *Weekly Farmers' Budget*. So, it looked good.

We selected for our victim the only child of a prominent citizen named Ebenezer Dorset. The father was respectable and tight, a mortgage fancier and a stern, upright collection-plate passer and forecloser. The kid was a boy of ten, with bas-relief freckles, and hair the colour of the cover of the magazine you buy at the news-stand when you want to catch a train. Bill and me figured that Ebenezer would melt down for a ransom of two thousand dollars to a cent. But wait till I tell you.

About two miles from Summit was a little mountain, covered with a dense cedar brake. On the rear elevation of this mountain was a cave. There we stored provisions. One evening after sundown, we drove in a buggy past old Dorset's house. The kid was in the street, throwing rocks at a kitten on the opposite fence.

"Hey, little boy!" says Bill, "would you like to have a bag of candy and a nice ride?"

The boy catches Bill neatly in the eye with a piece of brick.

"That will cost the old man an extra five hundred dollars," says Bill, climbing over the wheel.

That boy put up a fight like a welter-weight cinnamon bear; but, at last, we got him down in the bottom of the buggy and drove away. We took him up to the cave and I hitched the horse in the cedar brake. After dark I drove the buggy to the little village, three miles away, where we had hired it, and walked back to the mountain.

Bill was pasting court-plaster over the scratches and bruises on his features. There was a fire burning behind the big rock at the entrance of the cave, and the boy was watching a pot of boiling coffee, with two buzzard tail-feathers stuck in his red hair. He points a stick at me when I come up, and says:

"Ha! cursed paleface, do you dare to enter the camp of Red Chief, the terror of the plains?"

"He's all right now," says Bill, rolling up his trousers and examining some bruises on his shins. "We're playing Indian. We're making Buffalo Bill's show look like magic-lantern views of Palestine in the town hall. I'm Old Hank, the Trapper, Red Chief's captive, and I'm to be scalped at daybreak. By Geronimo! that kid can kick hard."

Yes, sir, that boy seemed to be having the time of his life. The fun of camping out in a cave had made him forget that he was a captive himself. He immediately christened me Snake-eye, the Spy, and announced that, when his braves returned from the warpath, I was to be broiled at the stake at the rising of the sun.

Then we had supper; and he filled his mouth full of bacon and bread and gravy, and began to talk. He made a during-dinner speech something like this:

"I like this fine. I never camped out before; but I had a pet 'possum once, and I was nine last birthday. I hate to go to school. Rats ate up sixteen of Jimmy Talbot's aunt's speckled hen's eggs. Are there any real Indians in these woods? I want some more gravy. Does the trees moving make the wind blow? We had five puppies. What makes your nose so red, Hank? My father has lots of money. Are the stars hot? I whipped Ed Walker twice, Saturday. I don't like girls. You dassent catch toads unless with a string. Do oxen make any noise? Why are oranges round? Have you got beds to sleep on in this cave? Amos Murray has got six toes. A parrot can talk, but a monkey or a fish can't. How many does it take to make twelve?"

Every few minutes he would remember that he was a pesky redskin, and pick up his stick rifle and tiptoe to the mouth of the cave to rubber for the scouts of the hated paleface. Now and then he would let out a war-whoop that made Old Hank the Trapper shiver. That boy had Bill terrorized from the start.

"Red Chief," says I to the kid, "would you like to go home?"

"Aw, what for?" says he. "I don't have any fun at home. I hate to go to school. I like to camp out. You won't take me back home again, Snake-eye, will you?"

"Not right away," says I. "We'll stay here in the cave a while."

"All right!" says he. "That'll be fine. I never had such fun in all my life."

We went to bed about eleven o'clock. We spread down some wide blankets and quilts and put Red Chief between us. We weren't afraid he'd run away. He kept us awake for three hours, jumping up and reaching for his rifle and screeching: "Hist! pard," in mine and Bill's ears, as the fancied crackle of a twig or the rustle of a leaf revealed to his young imagination the stealthy approach of the outlaw band. At last, I fell into a troubled sleep, and dreamed that I had been kidnapped and chained to a tree by a ferocious pirate with red hair.

Just at daybreak, I was awakened by a series of awful screams from Bill. They weren't yells, or howls, or shouts, or whoops, or yawps, such as you'd expect from a manly set of vocal organs—they were simply indecent, terrifying, humiliating screams, such as women emit when they see ghosts or caterpillars. It's an awful thing to hear a strong, desperate, fat man scream incontinently in a cave at daybreak.

I jumped up to see what the matter was. Red Chief was sitting on Bill's chest, with one hand twined in Bill's hair. In the other he had the sharp case-knife we used for slicing bacon; and he was industriously and realistically trying to take Bill's scalp, according to the sentence that had been pronounced upon him the evening before.

I got the knife away from the kid and made him lie down again. But, from that moment, Bill's spirit was broken. He laid down on his side of the bed, but he never closed an eye again in sleep as long as that boy was with us. I dozed off for a while, but along toward sun-up I remembered that Red Chief had said I was to be burned at the stake at the rising of the sun. I wasn't nervous or afraid; but I sat up and lit my pipe and leaned against a rock.

"What you getting up so soon for, Sam?" asked Bill.

"Me?" says I. "Oh, I got a kind of a pain in my shoulder. I thought sitting up would rest it."

"You're a liar!" says Bill. "You're afraid. You was to be burned at sunrise, and you was afraid he'd do it. And he would, too, if he could find a match. Ain't it awful, Sam? Do you think anybody will pay out money to get a little imp like that back home?"

"Sure," said I. "A rowdy kid like that is just the kind that parents dote on. Now, you and the Chief get up and cook breakfast, while I go up on the top of this mountain and reconnoitre."

I went up on the peak of the little mountain and ran my eye over the contiguous vicinity. Over toward Summit I expected to see the sturdy yeomanry of the village armed with scythes and pitchforks beating the countryside for the dastardly kidnappers. But what I saw was a peaceful landscape dotted with one man ploughing with a dun mule. Nobody was dragging the creek; no couriers dashed hither and yon, bringing tidings of no news to the distracted parents. There was a sylvan attitude of somnolent sleepiness pervading that section of the external outward surface of Alabama that lay exposed to my view. "Perhaps," says I to myself, "it has not yet been discovered that the wolves have borne away the tender lambkin from the fold. Heaven help the wolves!" says I, and I went down the mountain to breakfast.

When I got to the cave I found Bill backed up against the side of it, breathing hard, and the boy threatening to smash him with a rock half as big as a cocoanut.

"He put a red-hot boiled potato down my back," explained Bill, "and then mashed it with his foot; and I boxed his ears. Have you got a gun about you, Sam?"

I took the rock away from the boy and kind of patched up the argument. "I'll fix you," says the kid to Bill. "No man ever yet struck the Red Chief but what he got paid for it. You better beware!"

After breakfast the kid takes a piece of leather with strings wrapped around it out of his pocket and goes outside the cave unwinding it.

"What's he up to now?" says Bill, anxiously. "You don't think he'll run away, do you, Sam?"

"No fear of it," says I. "He don't seem to be much of a home body. But we've got to fix up some plan about the ransom. There don't seem to be much excitement around Summit on account of his disappearance; but maybe they haven't realized yet that he's gone. His folks may think he's spending the night with Aunt Jane or one of the neighbours. Anyhow, he'll be missed to-day. To-night we must get a message to his father demanding the two thousand dollars for his return."

Just then we heard a kind of war-whoop, such as David might have emitted when he knocked out the champion Goliath. It was a sling that Red Chief had pulled out of his pocket, and he was whirling it around his head.

I dodged, and heard a heavy thud and a kind of a sigh from Bill, like a horse gives out when you take his saddle off. A rock the size of an egg had caught Bill just behind his left ear. He loosened himself all over and fell in the fire across the frying pan of hot water for washing the dishes. I dragged him out and poured cold water on his head for half an hour.

By and by, Bill sits up and feels behind his ear and says: "Sam, do you know who my favourite Biblical character is?"

"Take it easy," says I. "You'll come to your senses presently."

"King Herod," says he. "You won't go away and leave me here alone, will you, Sam?"

I went out and caught that boy and shook him until his freckles rattled.

"If you don't behave," says I, "I'll take you straight home. Now, are you going to be good, or not?"

"I was only funning," says he sullenly. "I didn't mean to hurt Old Hank. But what did he hit me for? I'll behave, Snake-eye, if you won't send me home, and if you'll let me play the Black Scout to-day."

"I don't know the game," says I. "That's for you and Mr. Bill to decide. He's your playmate for the day. I'm going away for a while, on business. Now, you come in and make friends with him and say you are sorry for hurting him, or home you go, at once."

I made him and Bill shake hands, and then I took Bill aside and told him I was going to Poplar Cove, a little village three miles from the cave, and find out what I could about how the kidnapping had been regarded in Summit. Also, I thought it best to send a peremptory letter to old man Dorset that day, demanding the ransom and dictating how it should be paid.

"You know, Sam," says Bill, "I've stood by you without batting an eye in earthquakes, fire and flood—in poker games, dynamite outrages, police raids, train robberies and cyclones. I never lost my nerve yet till we kidnapped that two-legged skyrocket of a kid. He's got me going. You won't leave me long with him, will you, Sam?"

"I'll be back some time this afternoon," says I. "You must keep the boy amused and quiet till I return. And now we'll write the letter to old Dorset."

Bill and I got paper and pencil and worked on the letter while Red Chief, with a blanket wrapped around him, strutted up and down, guarding the mouth of the cave. Bill begged me tearfully to make the ransom fifteen hundred dollars instead of two thousand. "I ain't attempting," says he, "to decry the celebrated moral aspect of parental affection, but we're dealing with humans, and it ain't human for anybody to give up two thousand dollars for that forty-pound chunk of freckled wildcat. I'm willing to take a chance at fifteen hundred dollars. You can charge the difference up to me."

So, to relieve Bill, I acceded, and we collaborated a letter that ran this way:

Ebenezer Dorset, Esq.:

We have your boy concealed in a place far from Summit. It is useless for you or the most skilful detectives to attempt to find him. Absolutely, the only terms on which you can have him restored to you are these: We demand fifteen hundred dollars in large bills for his return; the money to be left at midnight to-night at the same spot and in the same box as your reply—as hereinafter described. If you agree to these terms, send your answer in writing by a solitary messenger to-night at half-past eight o'clock. After crossing Owl Creek, on the road to Poplar Cove, there are three large trees about

*a hundred yards apart, close to the fence of the wheat
field on the right-hand side. At the bottom of the fence-
post, opposite the third tree, will be found a small
pasteboard box.*

*The messenger will place the answer in this box and
return immediately to Summit.*

*If you attempt any treachery or fail to comply with
our demand as stated, you will never see your boy again.*

*If you pay the money as demanded, he will be
returned to you safe and well within three hours. These
terms are final, and if you do not accede to them no
further communication will be attempted.*

TWO DESPERATE MEN.

I addressed this letter to Dorset, and put it in my
pocket. As I was about to start, the kid comes up to me
and says:

"Aw, Snake-eye, you said I could play the Black
Scout while you was gone."

"Play it, of course," says I. "Mr. Bill will play with
you. What kind of a game is it?"

"I'm the Black Scout," says Red Chief, "and I have
to ride to the stockade to warn the settlers that the
Indians are coming. I'm tired of playing Indian myself.
I want to be the Black Scout."

"All right," says I. "It sounds harmless to me. I guess
Mr. Bill will help you foil the pesky savages."

"What am I to do?" asks Bill, looking at the kid
suspiciously.

"You are the hoss," says Black Scout. "Get down on
your hands and knees. How can I ride to the stockade
without a hoss?"

"You'd better keep him interested," said I, "till we get
the scheme going. Loosen up."

Bill gets down on his all fours, and a look comes in his eye like a rabbit's when you catch it in a trap.

"How far is it to the stockade, kid?" he asks, in a husky manner of voice.

"Ninety miles," says the Black Scout. "And you have to hump yourself to get there on time. Whoa, now!"

The Black Scout jumps on Bill's back and digs his heels in his side.

"For Heaven's sake," says Bill, "hurry back, Sam, as soon as you can. I wish we hadn't made the ransom more than a thousand. Say, you quit kicking me or I'll get up and warm you good."

I walked over to Poplar Cove and sat around the post office and store, talking with the chawbacons that came in to trade. One whiskerando says that he hears Summit is all upset on account of Elder Ebenezer Dorset's boy having been lost or stolen. That was all I wanted to know. I bought some smoking tobacco, referred casually to the price of black-eyed peas, posted my letter surreptitiously and came away. The postmaster said the mail-carrier would come by in an hour to take the mail on to Summit.

When I got back to the cave Bill and the boy were not to be found. I explored the vicinity of the cave, and risked a yodel or two, but there was no response.

So I lighted my pipe and sat down on a mossy bank to await developments.

In about half an hour I heard the bushes rustle, and Bill wabbled out into the little glade in front of the cave. Behind him was the kid, stepping softly like a scout, with a broad grin on his face. Bill stopped, took off his hat and wiped his face with a red handkerchief. The kid stopped about eight feet behind him.

"Sam," says Bill, "I suppose you'll think I'm a renegade, but I couldn't help it. I'm a grown person with masculine proclivities and habits of self-defence, but there is a time when all systems of egotism and predominance fail. The boy is gone. I have sent him home. All is off. There was martyrs in old times," goes on Bill, "that suffered death rather than give up the particular graft they enjoyed. None of 'em ever was subjugated to such supernatural tortures as I have been. I tried to be faithful to our articles of depredation; but there came a limit."

"What's the trouble, Bill?" I asks him.

"I was rode," says Bill, "the ninety miles to the stockade, not barring an inch. Then, when the settlers was rescued, I was given oats. Sand ain't a palatable substitute. And then, for an hour I had to try to explain to him why there was nothin' in holes, how a road can run both ways and what makes the grass green. I tell you, Sam, a human can only stand so much. I takes him by the neck of his clothes and drags him down the mountain. On the way he kicks my legs black-and-blue from the knees down; and I've got to have two or three bites on my thumb and hand cauterized.

"But he's gone"—continues Bill—"gone home. I showed him the road to Summit and kicked him about eight feet nearer there at one kick. I'm sorry we lose the ransom; but it was either that or Bill Driscoll to the madhouse."

Bill is puffing and blowing, but there is a look of ineffable peace and growing content on his rose-pink features.

"Bill," says I, "there isn't any heart disease in your family, is there?"

"No," says Bill, "nothing chronic except malaria and accidents. Why?"

"Then you might turn around," says I, "and have a look behind you."

Bill turns and sees the boy, and loses his complexion and sits down plump on the round and begins to pluck aimlessly at grass and little sticks. For an hour I was afraid for his mind. And then I told him that my scheme was to put the whole job through immediately and that we would get the ransom and be off with it by midnight if old Dorset fell in with our proposition. So Bill braced up enough to give the kid a weak sort of a smile and a promise to play the Russian in a Japanese war with him is soon as he felt a little better.

I had a scheme for collecting that ransom without danger of being caught by counterplots that ought to commend itself to professional kidnappers. The tree under which the answer was to be left—and the money later on—was close to the road fence with big, bare fields on all sides. If a gang of constables should be watching for anyone to come for the note they could see him a long way off crossing the fields or in the road. But no, sirree! At half-past eight I was up in that tree as well hidden as a tree toad, waiting for the messenger to arrive.

Exactly on time, a half-grown boy rides up the road on a bicycle, locates the pasteboard box at the foot of the fence-post, slips a folded piece of paper into it and pedals away again back toward Summit.

I waited an hour and then concluded the thing was square. I slid down the tree, got the note, slipped along the fence till I struck the woods, and was back at the cave in another half an hour. I opened the note, got near the lantern and read it to Bill. It was written with a pen in a crabbed hand, and the sum and substance of it was this:

Two Desperate Men.

   Gentlemen: I received your letter to-day by post, in regard to the ransom you ask for the return of my son. I think you are a little high in your demands, and I hereby make you a counter-proposition, which I am inclined to believe you will accept. You bring Johnny home and pay me two hundred and fifty dollars in cash, and I agree to take him off your hands. You had better come at night, for the neighbours believe he is lost, and I couldn't be responsible for what they would do to anybody they saw bringing him back. Very respectfully,
   EBENEZER DORSET.

"Great pirates of Penzance!" says I; "of all the impudent—"

But I glanced at Bill, and hesitated. He had the most appealing look in his eyes I ever saw on the face of a dumb or a talking brute.

"Sam," says he, "what's two hundred and fifty dollars, after all? We've got the money. One more night of this kid will send me to a bed in Bedlam. Besides being a thorough gentleman, I think Mr. Dorset is a spendthrift for making us such a liberal offer. You ain't going to let the chance go, are you?"

"Tell you the truth, Bill," says I, "this little he ewe lamb has somewhat got on my nerves too. We'll take him home, pay the ransom and make our get-away."

We took him home that night. We got him to go by telling him that his father had bought a silver-mounted rifle and a pair of moccasins for him, and we were going to hunt bears the next day.

It was just twelve o'clock when we knocked at Ebenezer's front door. Just at the moment when I should have been abstracting the fifteen hundred dollars from the box under the tree, according to the original proposition, Bill was counting out two hundred and fifty dollars into Dorset's hand.

When the kid found out we were going to leave him at home he started up a howl like a calliope and fastened himself as tight as a leech to Bill's leg. His father peeled him away gradually, like a porous plaster.

"How long can you hold him?" asks Bill.

"I'm not as strong as I used to be," says old Dorset, "but I think I can promise you ten minutes."

"Enough," says Bill. "In ten minutes I shall cross the Central, Southern and Middle Western States, and be legging it trippingly for the Canadian border."

And, as dark as it was, and as fat as Bill was, and as good a runner as I am, he was a good mile and a half out of Summit before I could catch up with him.

One of Those Impossible Americans

"*N'avez-vous pas—*" she was bravely demanding of the clerk when she saw that the bulky American who was standing there helplessly dangling two flaming red silk stockings which a copiously coiffured young woman assured him were *bien chic* was edging nearer her. She was never so conscious of the truly American quality of her French as when a countryman was at hand. The French themselves had an air of "How marvellously you speak!" but fellow Americans listened superciliously in an "I can do better than that myself" manner which quite untied the Gallic twist in one's tongue. And so, feeling her French was being compared, not with mere French itself, but with an arrogant new American brand thereof, she moved a little around the corner of the counter and began again in lower voice:

"*Mais, n'avez—*"

"Say, Young Lady," a voice which adequately represented the figure broke in, "*you*, aren't French, are you?"

She looked up with what was designed for a haughty stare. But what is a haughty stare to do in the face of a broad grin? And because it was such a long time since a grin like that had been grinned at her it happened that the stare gave way to a dimple, and the dimple to a laughing: "Is it so bad as that?"

"Oh, not your French," he assured her. "You talk it just like the rest of them. In fact, I should say, if anything—a little more so. But do you know,"—confidentially—"I can just spot an American girl every time!"

"How?" she could not resist asking, and the modest black hose she was thinking of purchasing dangled against his gorgeous red ones in friendliest fashion.

"Well, Sir—I don't know. I don't think it can be the clothes,"—judicially surveying her.

"The clothes," murmured Virginia, "were bought in Paris."

"Well, you've got *me*. Maybe it's the way you wear 'em. Maybe it's 'cause you look as if you used to play tag with your brother. Something—anyhow—gives a fellow that 'By jove there's an American girl!' feeling when he sees you coming round the corner."

"But why—?"

"Lord—don't begin on *why*. You can say *why* to anything. Why don't the French talk English? Why didn't they lay Paris out at right angles? Now look here, Young Lady, for that matter—*why* can't you help me buy some presents for my wife? There'd be nothing wrong about it," he hastened to assure her, "because my wife's a mighty fine woman."

The very small American looked at the very large one. Now Virginia was a well brought up young woman. Her conversations with strange men had been confined to such things as, "Will you please tell me the nearest way to—?" but preposterously enough—she could not for the life of her have told why—frowning upon this huge American—fat was the literal word—who stood there with puckered-up face swinging the flaming hose would seem in the same shameful class with snubbing the little boy who confidently asked her what kind of ribbon to buy for his mother.

"Was it for your wife you were thinking of buying these red stockings?" she ventured.

"Sure. What do you think of 'em? Look as if they came from Paris all right, don't they?"

"Oh, they look as though they came from Paris, all right," Virginia repeated, a bit grimly. "But do you know"—this quite as to that little boy who might be buying the ribbon—"American women don't always care for all the things that look as if they came from Paris. Is your wife—does she care especially for red stockings?"

"Don't believe she ever had a pair in her life. That's why I thought it might please her."

Virginia looked down and away. There were times when dimples made things hard for one.

Then she said, with gentle gravity: "There are quite a number of women in America who don't care much for red stockings. It would seem too bad, wouldn't it, if after you got these clear home your wife should turn out to be one of those people? Now, I think these grey stockings are lovely. I'm sure any woman would love them. She could wear them with grey suede slippers and they would be so soft and pretty."

"Um—not very lively looking, are they? You see I want something to cheer her up. She—well she's not been very well lately and I thought something—oh something with a lot of *dash* in it, you know, would just fill the bill. But look here. We'll take both. Sure—that's the way out of it. If she don't like the red, she'll like the grey, and if she don't like the—You like the grey ones, don't you? Then here"—picking up two pairs of the handsomely embroidered grey stockings and handing them to the clerk—"One," holding up his thumb to denote one—"me,"—a vigorous pounding of the chest

33

signifying me. "One"—holding up his forefinger and pointing to the girl—"mademoiselle."

"Oh no—no—no!" cried Virginia, her face instantly the colour of the condemned stockings. Then, standing straight: "Certainly *not*."

"No? Just as you say," he replied good humouredly. "Like to have you have 'em. Seems as if strangers in a strange land oughtn't to stand on ceremony."

The clerk was bending forward holding up the stockings alluringly. "*Pour mademoiselle, n'est-ce-pas?*"

"*Mais—non!*" pronounced Virginia, with emphasis.

There followed an untranslatable gesture. "How droll!" shoulder and outstretched hands were saying. "If the kind gentleman *wishes* to give mademoiselle the *joli bas*—!"

His face had puckered up again. Then suddenly it unpuckered. "Tell you what you might do," he solved it. "Just take 'em along and send them to your mother. Now your mother might be real glad to have 'em."

Virginia stared. And then an awful thing happened. What she was thinking about was the letter she could send with the stockings. "Mother dear," she would write, "as I stood at the counter buying myself some stockings to-day along came a nice man—a stranger to me, but very kind and jolly—and gave me—"

There it was that the awful thing happened. Her dimple was showing—and at thought of its showing she could not keep it from showing! And how could she explain why it was showing without its going on showing? And how—?

But at that moment her gaze fell upon the clerk, who had taken the dimple as signal to begin putting the stockings in a box. The Frenchwoman's eyebrows soon put that dimple in its proper place. "And so the *petite*

Americaine was not too—oh, not *too*—" those French eyebrows were saying.

All in an instant Virginia was something quite different from a little girl with a dimple. "You are very kind," she was saying, and her mother herself could have done it no better, "but I am sure our little joke had gone quite far enough. I bid you good-morning". And with that she walked regally over to the glove counter, leaving red and grey and black hosiery to their own destinies.

"I loathe them when their eyebrows go up," she fumed. "Now *his* weren't going up—not even in his mind."

She could not keep from worrying about him. "They'll just 'do' him," she was sure. "And then laugh at him in the bargain. A man like that has no *business* to be let loose in a store all by himself."

And sure enough, a half hour later she came upon him up in the dress department. Three of them had gathered round to "do" him. They were making rapid headway, their smiling deference scantily concealing their amused contempt. The spectacle infuriated Virginia. "They just think they can *work* us!" she stormed. "They think we're *easy*. I suppose they think he's a *fool*. I just wish they could get him in a business deal! I just wish—!"

"I can assure you, sir," the English-speaking manager of the department was saying, "that this garment is a wonderful value. We are able to let you have it at so absurdly low a figure because—"

Virginia did not catch why it was they were able to let him have it at so absurdly low a figure, but she did see him wipe his brow and look helplessly around. "Poor *thing*," she murmured, almost tenderly, "he doesn't know what to do. He just *does* need somebody to look after him." She stood there looking at his back. He had a back a good deal like the back of her chum's father at home. Indeed there were various things about him suggested "home." Did one want one's own jeered at? One might see crudities one's self, but was one going to have supercilious outsiders coughing those sham coughs behind their hypocritical hands?

"For seven hundred francs," she heard the suave voice saying.

Seven hundred francs! Virginia's national pride, or, more accurately, her national rage, was lashed into action. It was with very red cheeks that the small American stepped stormily to the rescue of her countryman.

"Seven hundred francs for *that*?" she jeered, right in the face of the enraged manager and stiffening clerks. "Seven hundred francs—indeed! Last year's model—a hideous colour, and"—picking it up, running it through her fingers and tossing it contemptuously aside— "abominable stuff!"

"Gee, but I'm grateful to you!" he breathed, again wiping his brow. "You know, I was a little leery of it myself."

The manager, quivering with rage and glaring uglily, stepped up to Virginia. "May I ask—?"

But the fat man stepped in between—he was well qualified for that position. "Cut it out, partner. The young lady's a friend of *mine*—see? She's looking out for me—not you. I don't want your stuff, anyway." And taking Virginia serenely by the arm he walked away.

"This was no place to buy dresses," said she crossly.

"Well, I wish I knew where the places *were* to buy things," he replied, humbly, forlornly.

"Well, what do you want to buy?" demanded she, still crossly.

"Why, I want to buy some nice things for my wife. Something the real thing from Paris, you know. I came over from London on purpose. But Lord,"—again wiping his brow—"a fellow doesn't know where to *go*."

"Oh well," sighed Virginia, long-sufferingly, "I see I'll just have to take you. There doesn't seem any way out of it. It's evident you can't go *alone. Seven hundred francs!*"

"I suppose it was too much," he conceded meekly. "I tell you I *will* be grateful if you'll just stay by me a little while. I never felt so up against it in all my life."

"Now, a very nice thing to take one's wife from Paris," began Virginia didactically, when they reached the sidewalk, "is lace."

"L—ace? Um! Y—es, I suppose lace is all right. Still it never struck me there was anything so very *lively* looking about lace."

"'Lively looking' is not the final word in wearing apparel," pronounced Virginia in teacher-to-pupil manner. "Lace is always in good taste, never goes out of style, and all women care for it. I will take you to one of the lace shops."

"Very well," acquiesced he, truly chastened. "Here, let's get in this cab."

Virginia rode across the Seine looking like one pondering the destinies of nations. Her companion turned several times to address her, but it would have been as easy for a soldier to slap a general on the back. Finally she turned to him.

"Now when we get there," she instructed, "don't seem at all interested in things. Act—oh, bored, you know, and seeming to want to get me away. And when they tell the price, no matter what they say, just—well sort of groan and hold your head and act as though you are absolutely overcome at the thought of such an outrage."

"U—m. You have to do that here to get—lace?"

"You have to do that here to get *anything*—at the price you should get it. You, and people who go shopping the way you do, bring discredit upon the entire American nation."

"That so? Sorry. Never meant to do that. All right, Young Lady, I'll do the best I can. Never did act that way, but suppose I can, if the rest of them do."

"Groan and hold my head," she heard him murmuring as they entered the shop.

He proved an apt pupil. It may indeed be set down that his aptitude was their undoing. They had no sooner entered the shop than he pulled out his watch and uttered an exclamation of horror at the sight of the time. Virginia could scarcely look at the lace, so insistently did he keep waving the watch before her. His contempt for everything shown was open and emphatic. It was also articulate. Virginia grew nervous, seeing the real red showing through in the Frenchwoman's cheeks. And when the price was at last named—a price which made Virginia jubilant—there burst upon her outraged ears something between a jeer and a howl of rage, the whole of it terrifyingly done in the form of a groan; she looked at her companion to see him holding up his hands and wobbling his head as though it had been suddenly loosened from his spine, cast one look at the Frenchwoman—then fled, followed by her groaning compatriot.

"I didn't mean you to act like *that*!" she stormed.

"Why, I did just what you told me to! Seemed to me I was following directions to the letter. Don't think for a minute *I'm* going to bring discredit on the American nation! Not a bad scheme—taking out my watch that way, was it?"

"Oh, beautiful *scheme*. I presume you notice, however, that we have no lace."

They walked half a block in silence. "Now I'll take you to another shop," she then volunteered, in a turning the other cheek fashion, "and here please do nothing at all. Please just—sit."

"Sort of as if I was feeble-minded, eh?"

"Oh, don't *try* to look feeble-minded," she begged, alarmed at seeming to suggest any more parts; "just sit there—as if you were thinking of something very far away."

"Say, Young Lady, look here; this is very nice, being put on to the tricks of the trade, but the money end of it isn't cutting much ice, and isn't there any way you can just *buy* things—the way you do in Cincinnati? Can't you get their stuff without making a comic opera out of it?"

"No, you can't," spoke relentless Virginia; "not unless you want them to laugh and say 'Aren't Americans fools?' the minute the door is shut."

"Fools—eh? I'll show them a thing or two!"

"Oh, please show them nothing here! Please just—sit."

While employing her wiles to get for three hundred and fifty francs a yoke and scarf aggregating four hundred, she chanced to look at her American friend. Then she walked rapidly to the rear of the shop, buried her face in her handkerchief, and seemed making heroic efforts to sneeze. Once more he was following directions to the letter. Chin resting on hands, hands resting on stick, the huge American had taken on the beatific expression of a seventeen-year-old girl thinking of something "very far away." Virginia was long in mastering the sneeze.

On the sidewalk she presented him with the package of lace and also with what she regarded the proper thing in the way of farewell speech. She supposed it *was* hard for a man to go shopping alone; she could see how hard it would be for her own father; indeed it was seeing how difficult it would be for her father had impelled her to go with him, a stranger. She trusted his wife would like the lace; she thought it very nice, and a bargain. She was glad to have been of service to a fellow countryman who seemed in so difficult a position.

But he did not look as impressed as one to whom a farewell speech was being made should look. In fact, he did not seem to be hearing it. Once more, and in earnest this time, he appeared to be thinking of something very far away. Then all at once he came back, and it was in anything but a far-away voice he began, briskly: "Now look here, Young Lady, I don't doubt but this lace is great stuff. You say so, and I haven't seen man, woman or child on this side of the Atlantic knows as much as you do. I'm mighty grateful for the lace—don't you forget that, but just the same—well, now I'll tell you. I have a very special reason for wanting something a little livelier than lace. Something that seems to have Paris written on it in red letters—see? Now, where do you get the kind of hats you see some folks wearing, and where do you get the dresses—well, it's hard to describe 'em, but the kind they have in pictures marked 'Breezes from Paris'? You see—S-ay!—what do you think of *that*?"

"That" was in a window across the street. It was an opera cloak. He walked toward it, Virginia following.

"Now *there*," he turned to her, his large round face all aglow, "is what I want."

It was yellow; it was long; it was billowy; it was insistently and recklessly regal.

"That's the ticket!" he gloated.

"Of course," began Virginia, "I don't know anything about it. I am in a very strange position, not knowing what your wife likes or—or has. This is the kind of thing everything has to go *with* or one wouldn't—one couldn't—"

"Sure! Good idea. We'll just get everything to go with it."

"It's the sort of thing one doesn't see worn much outside of Paris—or New York. If one is—now my mother wouldn't care for that coat at all." Virginia took no little pride in that tactful finish.

"Can't sidetrack me!" he beamed. "I *want* it. Very thing I'm after, Young Lady."

"Well, of course you will have no difficulty in buying the coat without me," said she, as a dignified version of "I wash my hands of you." "You can do here as you said you wished to do, simply go in and pay what they ask. There would be no use trying to get it cheap. They would know that anyone who wanted it would"—she wanted to say "have more money than they knew what to do with," but contented herself with, "be able to pay for it."

But when she had finished she looked at him; at first she thought she wanted to laugh, and then it seemed that wasn't what she wanted to do after all. It was like saying to a small boy who was one beam over finding a tin horn: "Oh well, take the horn if you want to, but you can't haul your little red waggon while you're blowing the horn." There seemed something peculiarly inhuman

41

about taking the waggon just when he had found the horn. Now if the waggon were broken, then to take away the horn would leave the luxury of grief. But let not shadows fall upon joyful moments.

With the full ardour of her femininity she entered into the purchasing of the yellow opera cloak. They paid for that decorative garment the sum of two thousand five hundred francs. It seemed it was embroidered, and the lining was—anyway, they paid it.

And they took it with them. He was going to "take no chances on losing it." He was leaving Paris that night and held that during his stay he had been none too impressed with either Parisian speed or Parisian veracity.

Then they bought some "Breezes from Paris," a dress that would "go with" the coat. It was violet velvet, and contributed to the sense of doing one's uttermost; and hats—"the kind you see some folks wearing." One was the rainbow done into flowers, and the other the kind of black hat to outdo any rainbow. "If you could just give me some idea what type your wife is," Virginia was saying, from beneath the willow plumes. "Now you see this hat quite overpowers me. Do you think it will overpower her?"

"Guess not. Anyway, if it don't look right on her head she may enjoy having it around to look at."

Virginia stared out at him. The *oddest* man! As if a hat were any good at all if it didn't look right on one's head!

Upon investigation—though yielding to his taste she was still vigilant as to his interests—Virginia discovered a flaw in one of the plumes. The sylph in the trailing gown held volubly that it did not *fait rien*; the man with the open purse said he couldn't see that it figured much, but the small American held firm. That must be replaced by a perfect plume or they would not take the hat. And when she saw who was in command the sylph as volubly acquiesced that *naturellement* it must be *tout a fait* perfect. She would send out and get one that would be oh! so, so, *so* perfect. It would take half an hour.

"Tell you what we'll do," Virginia's friend proposed, opera cloak tight under one arm, velvet gown as tight under the other, "I'm tired—hungry—thirsty; feel like a ham sandwich—and something. I'm playing you out, too. Let's go out and get a bite and come back for the so, so, *so* perfect hat."

She hesitated. But he had the door open, and if he stood holding it that way much longer he was bound to drop the violet velvet gown. She did not want him to drop the velvet gown and furthermore, she *would* like a cup of tea. There came into her mind a fortifying thought about the relative deaths of sheep and lambs. If to be killed for the sheep were indeed no worse than being killed for the lamb, and if a cup of tea went with the sheep and nothing at all with the lamb—?

So she agreed. "There's a nice little tea-shop right round the corner. We girls often go there."

"Tea? Like tea? All right, then"—and he started manfully on.

But as she entered the tea-shop she was filled with keen sense of the desirableness of being slain for the lesser animal. For, cosily installed in their favourite corner, were "the girls."

Virginia had explained to these friends some three hours before that she could not go with them that after-noon as she must attend a musicale some friends of her mother's were giving. Being friends of her mother's, she expatiated, she would have to go.

Recollecting this, also for the first time remembering the musicale, she bowed with the *hauteur* of self-consciousness.

Right there her friend contributed to the tragedy of a sheep's death by dropping the yellow opera cloak. While he was stooping to pick it up the violet velvet gown slid backward and Virginia had to steady it until he could regain position. The staring in the corner gave way to tittering—and no dying sheep had ever held its head more haughtily.

The death of this particular sheep proved long and painful. The legs of Virginia's friend and the legs of the tea-table did not seem well adapted to each other. He towered like a human mountain over the dainty thing, twisting now this way and now that. It seemed Providence—or at least so much of it as was represented by the management of that shop—had never meant fat people to drink tea. The table was rendered further out of proportion by having a large box piled on either side of it.

Expansively, and not softly, he discoursed of these things. What did they think a fellow was to do with his *knees*? Didn't they sell tea enough to afford any decent chairs? Did all these women pretend to really *like* tea?

Virginia's sense of humour rallied somewhat as she viewed him eating the sandwiches. Once she had called them doll-baby sandwiches; now that seemed literal: tea-cups, *petit gateau*, the whole service gave the fancy of his sitting down to a tea-party given by a little girl for her dollies.

But after a time he fell silent, looking around the

room. And when he broke that pause his voice was different.

"These women here, all dressed so fine, nothing to do but sit around and eat this folderol, *they* have it easy—don't they?"

The bitterness in it, and a faint note of wistfulness, puzzled her. Certainly *he* had money.

"And the husbands of these women," he went on; "lots of 'em, I suppose, didn't always have so much. Maybe some of these women helped out in the early days when things weren't so easy. Wonder if the men ever think how lucky they are to be able to get it back at 'em?"

She grew more bewildered. Wasn't he "getting it back?" The money he had been spending that day!

"Young Lady," he said abruptly, "you must think I'm a queer one."

She murmured feeble protest.

"Yes, you must. Must wonder what I want with all this stuff, don't you?"

"Why, it's for your wife, isn't it?" she asked, startled.

"Oh yes, but you must wonder. You're a shrewd one, Young Lady; judging the thing by me, you must wonder."

Virginia was glad she was not compelled to state her theory. Loud and common and impossible were terms which had presented themselves, terms which she had fought with kind and good-natured and generous. Their purchases she had decided were to be used, not for a knock, but as a crashing pound at the door of the society of his town. For her part, Virginia hoped the door would come down.

"And if you knew that probably this stuff would never be worn at all, that ten to one it would never do

45

anything more than lie round on chairs—then you *would* think I was queer, wouldn't you?"

She was forced to admit that that would seem rather strange.

"Young Lady, I believe I'll tell you about it. Never do talk about it to hardly anybody, but I feel as if you and I were pretty well acquainted—we've been through so much together."

She smiled at him warmly; there was something so real about him when he talked that way.

But his look then frightened her. It seemed for an instant as though he would brush the tiny table aside and seize some invisible thing by the throat. Then he said, cutting off each word short: "Young Lady, what do you think of this? I'm worth more 'an a million dollars—and my wife gets up at five o'clock every morning to do washing and scrubbing."

"Oh, it's not that she *has* to," he answered her look, "but she *thinks* she has to. See? Once we were poor. For twenty years we were poor as dirt. Then she did have to do things like that. Then I struck it. Or rather, it struck me. Oil. Oil on a bit of land I had. I had just sense enough to make the most of it; one thing led to another—well, you're not interested in that end of it. But the fact is that now we're rich. Now she could have all the things that these women have—Lord A'mighty she could lay abed every day till noon if she wanted to! But—you see?—it *got* her—those hard, lonely, grinding years *took* her. She's"—he shrunk from the terrible word and faltered out—"her mind's not—"

There was a sobbing little flutter in Virginia's throat. In a dim way she was glad to see that the girls were going. She *could* not have them laughing at him—now.

"Well, you can about figure out how it makes me

feel," he continued, and looking into his face now it was as though the spirit redeemed the flesh. "You're smart. You can see it without my callin' your attention to it. Last time I went to see her I had just made fifty thousand on a deal. And I found her down on her knees thinking she was scrubbing the floor!"

Unconsciously Virginia's hand went out, following the rush of sympathy and understanding. "But can't they—restrain her?" she murmured.

"Makes her worse. Says she's got it to do—frets her to think she's not getting it done."

"But isn't there some *way*?" she whispered. "Some way to make her *know*?"

He pointed to the large boxes. "That," he said simply, "is the meaning of those. It's been seven years—but I keep on trying."

She was silent, the tears too close for words. And she had thought it cheap ambition!—vulgar aspiration— silly show—vanity!

"Suppose you thought I was a queer one, talking about lively looking things. But you see now? Thought it might attract her attention, thought something real gorgeous like this might impress money on her. Though I don't know,"—he seemed to grow weary as he told it; "I got her a lot of diamonds, thinking they might interest her, and she thought that she'd stolen 'em, and they had to take them away."

Still the girl did not speak. Her hand was shading her eyes.

"But there's nothing like trying. Nothing like keeping right on trying. And anyhow—a fellow likes to think he's taking his wife something from Paris."

They passed before her in their heartbreaking folly, their tragic uselessness, their lovable absurdity and

47

stinging irony—those things they had bought that after-noon: an *opera cloak*—a *velvet dress*—*those hats*—*red silk stockings*.

The mockery of them wrung her heart. Right there in the tea-shop Virginia was softly crying.

"Oh, now that's too bad," he expostulated clumsily. "Why, look here, Young Lady, I didn't mean you to take it so hard."

When she had recovered herself he told her much of the story. And the thing which revealed him—glorified him—was less the grief he gave to it than the way he saw it. "It's the cursed unfairness of it," he concluded. "When you consider it's all because she did those things—when you think of her bein' bound to 'em for life just because she was *too faithful doin' 'em*—when you think that now—when I could give her everything these women have got!—she's got to go right on worrying about baking the bread and washing the dishes—did it for me when I was poor—and now with me rich she can't get *out* of it—and I *can't reach* her—oh, it's rotten! I tell you it's *rotten*! Sometimes I can just hear my money *laugh* at me! Sometimes I get to going round and round in a circle about it till it seems I'm going crazy myself."

"I think you are a—a noble man," choked Virginia.

That disconcerted him. "Oh Lord—don't think that. No, Young Lady, don't try to make any plaster saint out of *me*. My life goes on. I've got to eat, drink and be merry. I'm built that way. But just the same my heart on the inside's pretty sore, Young Lady. I want to tell you that the whole inside of my heart is *sore as a boil*!"

They were returning for the hats. Suddenly Virginia stopped, and it was a soft-eyed and gentle Virginia who turned to him after the pause. "There are lovely things to be bought in Paris for women who aren't well. Such soft, lovely things to wear in your room. Not but what I think these other things are all right. As you say, they may—interest her. But they aren't things she can use just now, and wouldn't you like her to have some of those soft lovely things she could actually wear? They might help most of all. To wake in the morning and find herself in something so beautiful—"

"Where do you get 'em?" he demanded promptly.

And so they went to one of those shops which have, more than all the others, enshrined Paris in feminine hearts. And never was lingerie selected with more loving care than that which Virginia picked out that afternoon. A tear fell on one particularly lovely *robe de nuit*—so soothingly soft, so caressingly luxurious, it seemed that surely it might help bring release from the bondage of those crushing years.

As they were leaving they were given two packages. "Just the kimona thing you liked," he said, "and a trinket or two. Now that we're such good friends, you won't feel like you did this morning."

"And if I don't want them myself, I might send them to my mother," Virginia replied, a quiver in her laugh at her own little joke.

He had put her in her cab; he had tried to tell her how much he thanked her; they had said good-bye and the *cocher* had cracked his whip when he came running after her. "Why, Young Lady," he called out, "we don't know each other's *names*."

She laughed and gave hers. "Mine's William P. Johnson," he said. "Part French and part Italian. But now look here, Young Lady—or I mean, Miss Clayton. A fellow at the hotel was telling me something last night that made me *sick*. He said American girls sometimes

49

got awfully up against it here. He said one actually starved last year. Now, I don't like that kind of business. Look here, Young Lady, I want you to promise that if you—you or any of your gang—get up against it you'll cable William P. Johnson, of Cincinnati, Ohio."

The twilight grey had stolen upon Paris. And there was a mist which the street lights only penetrated a little way—as sometimes one's knowledge of life may only penetrate life a very little way. Her cab stopped by a blockade, she watched the burly back of William P. Johnson disappearing into the mist. The red box which held the yellow opera cloak she could see longer than all else.

"You never can tell," murmured Virginia. "It just goes to show that you never can tell."

And whatever it was you never could tell had brought to Virginia's girlish face the tender knowingness of the face of a woman.

Happiness

It was tea time—the hour before the lamps were brought in. The villa overlooked the sea; the sun had disappeared and left in its wake a crimson sky flecked with gold; and the Mediterranean, not a ripple disturbing its smooth, gleaming surface, looked like a polished and limitless sheet of metal.

To the right, in the far distance, jagged mountain peaks reared their dusky outline against the tender purple of the sunset.

The company were talking of love—that old, old theme—and were saying for the hundredth time things well known to them all. The gentle melancholy of twilight made their words slow and soft, their hearts more easily moved than usual; and the word "love," pronounced now in a man's firm voice, now in a woman's musical tones, held an unwonted glamour for them all. It seemed to fill the little drawing-room, to flutter, bird-like, through the air, to hover like a spirit above their heads.

"Can one's love last for years?"

"Yes," affirmed some.

"No," said others.

Cases were quoted, examples cited; and all the guests, men and women, full of recollections they could not reveal, which arose insistently in their minds, seemed profoundly moved, and spoke with hushed voices of that mystic, potent bond which unites man and woman for good or ill.

But suddenly someone who had been gazing out into the distance cried:

"Oh, look! Look! What is that?"

Above the sea there rose, on the horizon, a large, greyish, indeterminate mass.

The women stood up, and looked wonderingly at this unexpected object, which they had never before seen.

Someone said:

"That is Corsica! It is visible like that only two or three times in the year, under certain exceptional atmospheric conditions, when the air, being absolutely clear, does not conceal it behind those curtains of sea mist which usually veil the horizon."

The Corsican mountains were vaguely distinguishable; the gazers fancied they could even see the snow on their peaks. And all were surprised, moved, well-nigh alarmed, at this sudden apparition of a world rising, phantom-like, out of the sea. Perhaps they saw strange visions, like those which appeared to Columbus from beyond the unexplored, the unknown, ocean.

Presently an old man who had not yet spoken said:

"Stay! In that very island which appears before us now, as if to answer our question by recalling to my mind a long-banished memory, I once knew a wonderful example of constant love, of an enduring and supremely happy love. I will tell the story:

"Five years ago I went on a trip through Corsica. This semi-barbarous island is less known to us, and is in reality farther from us, than America; although, as is the case today, it can sometimes be seen from the French coast.

"Picture to yourself a still chaotic world, a wilderness

52

of mountains separated from one another by narrow valleys, through which rush swirling torrents; no plain, only immense waves of granite and huge undulations of the earth clothed with shrubs or with forests of lofty chestnut trees and pines. The soil is a virgin one, untilled, neglected, though here and there one comes across a village, looking like a pile of rocks, at the summit of a hill. The island boasts neither agriculture, industry, not art. Never does one see a piece of carved wood or a block of sculptured stone, or any testimony whatever to artistic taste on the part of the aborigines. It is just this which strikes one most in this superb yet ungracious land; hereditary indifference toward that striving after the beautiful in form which we call art.

"Italy, where every place, full of works of art, is itself a work of art; where marble, wood, bronze, iron, metals, and stones all testify to the genius of man; where the smallest object lying in ancient houses reveals a divine regard for grace of form—Italy is for us the well-beloved and sacred country, because she shows us and proves to us the greatness, the power, and the triumph of creative intelligence.

"And right opposite her, savage Corsica has remained what she was from the first. Her inhabitants dwell in their rough-hewn houses, indifferent to all that does not affect their actual existence or their family quarrels. And they have retained both the faults and the virtues of primitive races. They are violent, vindictive, blood-thirsty; but they are also simple, hospitable, generous, opening their doors to the passer-by, and rewarding with absolute fidelity the smallest mark of sympathy.

"Well, for a month I had been wandering through this magnificent island, with a kind of feeling that I had reached the end of the earth. No inns, no public houses,

no roads. You reach by mule paths those hamlets cling-
ing to the mountainside, where the never-ceasing roar of
the torrent below assails the ear from morning till night.
You knock at the door of a house; you a night's shelter
and enough food to last you till the following evening.
And you sit down at the humble board, you sleep under
the humble roof, and next morning you part, with a
hearty handshake, from your host, who has conducted
you as far as the end of the village.

"One evening, after ten hours on the road, I came
across a little dwelling standing by itself at the head of
a narrow valley which debouched on the sea some three
miles off. The two steep mountainsides, covered with
shrubs, boulders, and loft trees, were as two dark walls
shutting in this cheerless ravine.

"Round the cottage were a few vines, a small garden,
and one or two large chestnut trees. Here were the
means of subsistence, at all events—almost a fortune,
indeed, in this poverty-stricken land.

"The woman who received me was old, of austere
aspect, and—wonderful to relate—very clean. The man,
sitting on a rush-bottomed chair, rose in sign of welcome, and then sat down again without a word.

"'Please excuse him,' said his companion. 'He's quite
deaf. He's eighty-two years old.'

"She spoke the French of France. I was surprised.

"'You do not belong to Corsica?' I asked.

"'No,' she said; 'we are from the Continent; but we
have lived here for the last fifty years.'

"I shuddered at the thought of fifty years spent in
this God-forsaken spot, far from the haunts of men. An
old shepherd joined us, and we all sat down to the
single dish of which the dinner consisted—a thick soup

in which potatoes, bacon, and cabbage had been boiled together.

"When the brief meal was over I went and sat before the door, a prey to that melancholy which sometimes seizes travellers in certain lonely places or on certain lonely evenings. At such times one feels that everything is at an end—one's life, the very universe. One gets a sudden, fearful glimpse of the abject misery of life; the isolation of every human being from his fellows; the black, hopeless solitude of the heart, which, neverthe-less, cheats itself with dreams until the day of death.

"The old woman joined me, and, possessed with that curiosity which survives in even the most placid and resigned of mortals, said:

"'So you come from France?'

"'Yes. I am on a pleasure trip.'

"'You are from Paris, perhaps?'

"'No; I am from Nancy.'

"At this juncture the man, impassible like all deaf people, appeared in the doorway. She continued:

"'Never mind him; he can't hear.'

"Then, after a few moments' pause:

"'Do you know the people of Nancy?'

"'Yes; nearly everybody.'

"'The Sainte-Allaize family?'

"'Yes, very well; they are friends of my father.'

"'What is your name?'

"I told her. She looked at me fixedly, then murmured in a pensive tone, occasioned by the stirring of long-forgotten memories:

"'Yes, yes; I remember well. And what has become of the Brismares?'

"'They are all dead.'

"'Ah! And did you know the Sirmonts?'

"'Yes; the last of them is a general.'

"Then she said, trembling with emotion and moved by an irresistible impulse to confess, to tell all, to speak of those things which had hitherto remained locked in her own bosom, and of those people whose name affected her beyond words:

"'Yes; Henri de Sirmont. I know him; he is my brother.'

"I raised my eyes to her, speechless with astonishment. And suddenly I remembered.

"There had long ago been a great scandal in the Sirmont family. Suzanne de Sirmont, young, beautiful, and rich, eloped with a non-commissioned officer in the regiment of hussars her father commanded.

"He was a handsome man of peasant birth, a man who looked well in his uniform—this soldier who had seduced his colonel's daughter. She had, no doubt, seen him, singled him out, and fallen in love with him, when watching her father's squadrons file by. But how had she got speech with him? How had they managed to see each other and come to an understanding? No one ever knew.

"Such a catastrophe had never been dreamed of. One evening the soldier disappeared with her. Search was made, but the pair were never discovered. No news of them was ever received, and Suzanne de Sirmont was looked upon as dead.

"And now I had discovered her in this gloomy valley!

" Then I asked in my turn:

"'Yes; I remember. You are Mademoiselle Suzanne?'

"She nodded her head in sign of assent. Tears fell from her eyes. Then, pointing to the old man framed in the doorway, she said:

"'That is he.'

56

"And I saw that she still loved him, that she still looked at him with the eyes of affection.

"'Have you been happy?' I asked.

"'Oh, yes,' she replied in a voice that came straight from her heart; 'very happy. He has made me perfectly happy. I have never had a moment's regret.'

"I looked at her, astonished at this exhibition of the power of love. Here was a rich girl who had followed a mere peasant. She had become a peasant herself. She had resigned herself to a life destitute of charm, of luxury, of refinement of any sort; she had accommodated herself to her husband's simple ways. And she still loved him. She had become a woman of the people, wearing a cap and a coarse stiff skirt. She ate her food off an earthenware plate, on a rough wooden table, sitting on a rush-bottomed chair. Her dinner consisted of cabbage and potato soup. She lay on a hard mattress at his side.

"And she had never thought of anything but him! She had not regretted her jewels, her clothes, all the elegances of her toilet, the softness of her chairs, the perfumed warmth of her curtained boudoir, the downy softness of her bed. She had never needed aught but him; if he were there she desired nothing more.

"She had, when quite young, forsaken her life, the world, and all those who had brought her up and loved her. She had come, alone with him, to this desolate valley. And he had been everything to her—her hopes, her dreams, her desires. He had filled her whole existence with contentment.

"She could not have been happier.

"And all night long, listening to the harsh breathing of the old solider, extended on his pallet beside her who had followed him so far, I thought of their story, strange in its simplicity; of their happiness, so complete, yet made up of so little."

The narrator was silent. A woman said:

"But she had too lowly an ideal. Her needs were too simple, her instincts too primitive. She must have been a weak sort of creature."

Another said slowly:

"What matter! She was happy."

And on the far-off horizon Corsica melted into the grey night, was slowly swallowed up by the sea, withdrew that shadowy outline which had risen up as if to tell the story of the two humble lovers its rugged shores had sheltered.

LAURA E. RICHARDS

The Golden Windows

All day long the little boy worked hard, in field and barn and shed, for his people were poor farmers, and could not pay a workman; but at sunset there came an hour that was all his own, for his father had given it to him. Then the boy would go up to the top of a hill and look across at another hill that rose some miles away. On this far hill stood a house with windows of clear gold and diamonds. They shone and blazed so that it made the boy wink to look at them: but after a while the people in the house put up shutters, as it seemed, and then it looked like any common farmhouse. The boy supposed they did this because it was supper-time; and then he would go into the house and have his supper of bread and milk, and so to bed.

One day the boy's father called him and said: "You have been a good boy, and have earned a holiday. Take this day for your own; but remember that God gave it, and try to learn some good thing."

The boy thanked his father and kissed his mother; then he put a piece of bread in his pocket, and started off to find the house with the golden windows.

It was pleasant walking. His bare feet made marks in the white dust, and when he looked back, the footprints seemed to be following him, and making company for him. His shadow, too, kept beside him, and would dance or run with him as he pleased; so it was very cheerful.

By and by he felt hungry; and he sat down by a

59

brown brook that ran through the alder hedge by the roadside, and ate his bread, and drank the clear water. Then he scattered the crumbs for the birds, as his mother had taught him to do, and went on his way.

After a long time he came to a high green hill; and when he had climbed the hill, there was the house on the top; but it seemed that the shutters were up, for he could not see the golden windows. He came up to the house, and then he could well have wept, for the windows were of clear glass, like any others, and there was no gold anywhere about them.

A woman came to the door, and looked kindly at the boy, and asked him what he wanted.

"I saw the golden windows from our hilltop," he said, "and I came to see them, but now they are only glass."

The woman shook her head and laughed.

"We are poor farming people," she said, "and are not likely to have gold about our windows; but glass is better to see through."

She bade the boy sit down on the broad stone step at the door, and brought him a cup of milk and a cake, and bade him rest; then she called her daughter, a child of his own age, and nodded kindly at the two, and went back to her work.

The little girl was barefooted like himself, and wore a brown cotton gown, but her hair was golden like the windows he had seen, and her eyes were blue like the sky at noon. She led the boy about the farm, and showed him her black calf with the white star on its forehead, and he told her about his own at home, which was red like a chestnut, with four white feet. Then when they had eaten an apple together, and so had become friends, the boy asked her about the golden windows.

The little girl nodded, and said she knew all about them, only he had mistaken the house.

"You have come quite the wrong way!" she said. "Come with me, and I will show you the house with the golden windows, and then you will see for yourself."

They went to a knoll that rose behind the farmhouse, and as they went the little girl told him that the golden windows could only be seen at a certain hour, about sunset.

"Yes, I know that!" said the boy.

When they reached the top of the knoll, the girl turned and pointed; and there on a hill far away stood a house with windows of clear gold and diamond, just as he had seen them. And when they looked again, the boy saw that it was his own home.

Then he told the little girl that he must go; and he gave her his best pebble, the white one with the red band, that he had carried for a year in his pocket; and she gave him three horse-chestnuts, one red like satin, one spotted, and one white like milk. He kissed her, and promised to come again, but he did not tell her what he had learned; and so he went back down the hill, and the little girl stood in the sunset light and watched him.

The way home was long, and it was dark before the boy reached his father's house; but the lamplight and firelight shone through the windows, making them almost as bright as he had seen them from the hilltop; and when he opened the door, his mother came to kiss him, and his little sister ran to throw her arms about his neck, and his father looked up and smiled from his seat by the fire.

"Have you had a good day?" asked his mother.

Yes, the boy had had a very good day.

"And have you learned anything?" asked his father.

"Yes!" said the boy. "I have learned that our house has windows of gold and diamond."

H. G. WELLS

The Man Who Could Work Miracles

It is doubtful whether the gift was innate. For my own part, I think it came to him suddenly. Indeed, until he was thirty he was a sceptic, and did not believe in miraculous powers. And here, since it is the most convenient place, I must mention that he was a little man, and had eyes of a hot brown, very erect red hair, a moustache with ends that he twisted up, and freckles. His name was George McWhirter Fotheringay—not the sort of name by any means to lead to any expectation of miracles—and he was clerk at Gomshott's. He was greatly addicted to assertive argument. It was while he was asserting the impossibility of miracles that he had his first intimation of his extraordinary powers. This particular argument was being held in the bar of the Long Dragon, and Toddy Beamish was conducting the opposition by a monotonous but effective "So *you* say," that drove Mr. Fotheringay to the very limit of his patience.

There were present, besides these two, a very dusty cyclist, landlord Cox, and Miss Maybridge, the perfectly respectable and rather portly barmaid of the Dragon. Miss Maybridge was standing with her back to Mr. Fotheringay, washing glasses; the others were watching him, more or less amused by the present ineffectiveness of the assertive method. Goaded by the Torres Vedras tactics of Mr. Beamish, Mr. Fotheringay determined to make an unusual rhetorical effort.

"Looky here, Mr. Beamish," said Mr. Fotheringay. "Let us clearly understand what a miracle is. It's something contrariwise to the course of nature done by power of Will, something what couldn't happen without being specially willed."

"So *you* say," said Mr. Beamish, repulsing him.

Mr. Fotheringay appealed to the cyclist, who had hitherto been a silent auditor, and received his assent—given with a hesitating cough and a glance at Mr. Beamish. The landlord would express no opinion, and Mr. Fotheringay, returning to Mr. Beamish, received the unexpected concession of a qualified assent to his definition of a miracle.

"For instance," said Mr. Fotheringay, greatly encouraged. "Here would be a miracle. That lamp, in the natural course of nature, couldn't burn like that upsy-down, could it, Beamish?"

"*You* say it couldn't," said Beamish.

"And you?" said Fotheringay. "You don't mean to say—eh?"

"No," said Beamish reluctantly. "No, it couldn't."

"Very well," said Mr. Fotheringay. "Then here comes someone, as it might be me, along here, and stands as it might be here, and says to that lamp, as I might do, collecting all my will—Turn upsy-down without breaking, and go on burning steady, and—Hullo!"

It was enough to make anyone say "Hullo!" The impossible, the incredible, was visible to them all. The lamp hung inverted in the air, burning quietly with its flame pointing down. It was as solid, as indisputable as ever a lamp was, the prosaic common lamp of the Long Dragon bar.

Mr. Fotheringay stood with an extended forefinger and the knitted brows of one anticipating a catastrophic smash. The cyclist, who was sitting next the lamp, ducked and jumped across the bar. Everybody jumped, more or less. Miss Maybridge turned and screamed. For nearly three seconds the lamp remained still. A faint cry of mental distress came from Mr. Fotheringay. "I can't keep it up," he said, "any longer." He staggered back, and the inverted lamp suddenly flared, fell against the corner of the bar, bounced aside, smashed upon the floor, and went out.

It was lucky it had a metal receiver, or the whole place would have been in a blaze. Mr. Cox was the first to speak, and his remark, shorn of needless excrescences, was to the effect that Fotheringay was a fool. Fotheringay was beyond disputing even so fundamental a proposition as that! He was astonished beyond measure at the thing that had occurred. The subsequent conversation threw absolutely no light on the matter so far as Fotheringay was concerned; the general opinion not only followed Mr. Cox very closely but very vehemently. Everyone accused Fotheringay of a silly trick, and presented him to himself as a foolish destroyer of comfort and security. His mind was in a tornado of perplexity, he was himself inclined to agree with them, and he made a remarkably ineffectual opposition to the proposal of his departure.

He went home flushed and heated, coat-collar crumpled, eyes smarting and ears red. He watched each of the ten street lamps nervously as he passed it. It was only when he found himself alone in his little bed-room in Church Row that he was able to grapple seriously with his memories of the occurrence, and ask, "What on earth happened?"

He had removed his coat and boots, and was sitting on the bed with his hands in his pockets repeating the text of his defence for the seventeenth time, "*I* didn't want the confounded thing to upset," when it occurred to him that at the precise moment he had said the commanding words he had inadvertently willed the thing he said, and that when he had seen the lamp in the air he had felt that it depended on him to maintain it there without being clear how this was to be done. He had not a particularly complex mind, or he might have stuck for a time at that "inadvertently willed," embracing, as it does, the abstrusest problems of voluntary action; but as it was, the idea came to him with a quite acceptable haziness. And from that, following, as I must admit, no clear logical path, he came to the test of experiment.

He pointed resolutely to his candle and collected his mind, though he felt he did a foolish thing. "Be raised up," he said. But in a second that feeling vanished. The candle was raised, hung in the air one giddy moment, and as Mr. Fotheringay gasped, fell with a smash on his toilet-table, leaving him in darkness save for the expiring glow of its wick.

For a time Mr. Fotheringay sat in the darkness, perfectly still. "It did happen, after all," he said. "And 'ow I'm to explain it I *don't* know." He sighed heavily, and began feeling in his pockets for a match. He could find none, and he rose and groped about the toilet-table. "I wish I had a match," he said. He resorted to his coat, and there was none there, and then it dawned upon him that miracles were possible even with matches. He extended a hand and scowled at it in the dark. "Let there be a match in that hand," he said. He felt some light object fall across his palm, and his fingers closed upon a match.

After several ineffectual attempts to light this, he

discovered it was a safety-match. He threw it down, and then it occurred to him that he might have willed it lit. He did, and perceived it burning in the midst of his toilet-table mat. He caught it up hastily, and it went out. His perception of possibilities enlarged, and he felt for and replaced the candle in its candlestick. "Here! *you* be lit," said Mr. Fotheringay, and forthwith the candle was flaring, and he saw a little black hole in the toilet-cover, with a wisp of smoke rising from it. For a time he stared from this to the little flame and back, and then looked up and met his own gaze in the looking glass. By this help he communed with himself in silence for a time.

"How about miracles now?" said Mr. Fotheringay at last, addressing his reflection.

The subsequent meditations of Mr. Fotheringay were of a severe but confused description. So far, he could see it was a case of pure willing with him. The nature of his experiences so far disinclined him for any further experiments, at least until he had reconsidered them. But he lifted a sheet of paper, and turned a glass of water pink and then green, and he created a snail, which he miraculously annihilated, and got himself a miraculous new tooth-brush. Somewhere in the small hours he had reached the fact that his will-power must be of a particularly rare and pungent quality, a fact of which he had certainly had inklings before, but no certain assurance. The scare and perplexity of his first discovery was now qualified by pride in this evidence of singularity and by vague intimations of advantage. He became aware that the church clock was striking one, and as it did not occur to him that his daily duties at Gomshott's might be miraculously dispensed with, he resumed undressing, in order to get to bed without further delay. As he struggled to get his shirt over his head, he was struck with a brilliant idea. "Let me be in bed," he said, and found himself so. "Undressed," he stipulated; and, finding the sheets cold, added hastily, "and in my nightshirt—no, in a nice soft woollen nightshirt. Ah!" he said with immense enjoyment. "And now let me be comfortably asleep . . ."

He awoke at his usual hour and was pensive all through breakfast-time, wondering whether his overnight experience might not be a particularly vivid dream. At length his mind turned again to cautious experiments. For instance, he had three eggs for breakfast; two his landlady had supplied, good, but shoppy, and one was a delicious fresh goose-egg, laid, cooked, and served by his extraordinary will. He hurried off to Gomshott's in a state of profound but carefully concealed excitement, and only remembered the shell of the third egg when his landlady spoke of it that night. All day he could do no work because of this astonishingly new self-knowledge, but this caused him no inconvenience, because he made up for it miraculously in his last ten minutes.

As the day wore on his state of mind passed from wonder to elation, albeit the circumstances of his dismissal from the Long Dragon were still disagreeable to recall, and a garbled account of the matter that had reached his colleagues led to some badinage. It was evident he must be careful how he lifted frangible articles, but in other ways his gift promised more and more as he turned it over in his mind. He intended among other things to increase his personal property by unostentatious acts of creation. He called into existence a pair of very splendid diamond studs, and hastily annihilated them again as young Gomshott came across the counting-house to his desk. He was afraid young Gom-shott might wonder how he had come by them. He saw quite clearly the gift required caution and watchfulness in its exercise, but so far as he could judge the difficulties attending its mastery would be no greater than those he had already faced in the study of cycling. It was that analogy, perhaps, quite as much as the feeling that he would be unwelcome in the Long Dragon, that drove him out after supper into the lane beyond the gas-works, to rehearse a few miracles in private.

There was possibly a certain want of originality in his attempts, for apart from his will-power Mr. Fotheringay was not a very exceptional man. The miracle of Moses' rod came to his mind, but the night was dark and unfavourable to the proper control of large miraculous snakes. Then he recollected the story of "Tannhäuser" that he had read on the back of the Philharmonic programme. That seemed to him singularly attractive and harmless. He stuck his walking-stick—a very nice Poona-Penang lawyer—into the turf that edged the footpath, and commanded the dry wood to blossom. The air was immediately full of the scent of roses, and by means of a match he saw for himself that this beautiful miracle was indeed accomplished. His satisfaction was ended by advancing footsteps. Afraid of a premature discovery of his powers, he addressed the blossoming stick hastily: "Go back." What he meant was "Change back;" but of course he was confused. The stick receded at a considerable velocity, and incontinently came a cry of anger and a bad word from the approaching person. "Who are you throwing brambles at, you fool?" cried a voice. "That got me on the shin."

"I'm sorry, old chap," said Mr. Fotheringay, and

then realising the awkward nature of the explanation, caught nervously at his moustache. He saw Winch, one of the three Immering constables, advancing.

"What d'yer mean by it?" asked the constable. "Hullo! It's you, is it? The gent that broke the lamp at the Long Dragon!"

"I don't mean anything by it," said Mr. Fotheringay. "Nothing at all."

"What d'yer do it for then?"

"Oh, bother!" said Mr. Fotheringay.

"Bother indeed! D'yer know that stick hurt? What d'yer do it for, eh?"

For the moment Mr. Fotheringay could not think what he had done it for. His silence seemed to irritate Mr. Winch. "You've been assaulting the police, young man, this time. That's what *you* done."

"Look here, Mr. Winch," said Mr. Fotheringay, annoyed and confused, "I'm very sorry. The fact is—"

"Well?"

He could think of no way but the truth. "I was working a miracle." He tried to speak in an off-hand way, but try as he would he couldn't.

"Working a—! 'Ere, don't you talk rot. Working a miracle, indeed! Miracle! Well, that's downright funny! Why, you's the chap that don't believe in miracles . . . Fact is, this is another of your silly conjuring tricks—that's what this is. Now, I tell you—"

But Mr. Fotheringay never heard what Mr. Winch was going to tell him. He realised he had given himself away, flung his valuable secret to all the winds of heaven. A violent gust of irritation swept him to action. He turned on the constable swiftly and fiercely. "Here," he said, "I've had enough of this, I have! I'll show you a silly conjuring trick, I will! Go to Hades! Go, now!"

He was alone!

Mr. Fotheringay performed no more miracles that night, nor did he trouble to see what had become of his flowering stick. He returned to the town, scared and very quiet, and went to his bed-room. "Lord!" he said, "it's a powerful gift—an extremely powerful gift. I didn't hardly mean as much as that. Not really . . . I wonder what Hades is like!"

He sat on the bed taking off his boots. Struck by a happy thought he transferred the constable to San Francisco, and without any more interference with normal causation went soberly to bed. In the night he dreamt of the anger of Winch.

The next day Mr. Fotheringay heard two interesting items of news. Someone had planted a most beautiful climbing rose against the elder Mr. Gomshott's private house in the Lullaborough Road, and the river as far as Rawling's Mill was to be dragged for Constable Winch.

Mr. Fotheringay was abstracted and thoughtful all that day, and performed no miracles except certain provisions for Winch, and the miracle of completing his day's work with punctual perfection in spite of all the bee-swarm of thoughts that hummed through his mind. And the extraordinary abstraction and meekness of his manner was remarked by several people, and made a matter for jesting. For the most part he was thinking of Winch.

On Sunday evening he went to chapel, and oddly enough, Mr. Maydig, who took a certain interest in occult matters, preached about "things that are not lawful." Mr. Fotheringay was not a regular chapel goer, but the system of assertive scepticism, to which I have already alluded, was now very much shaken. The tenor of the sermon threw an entirely new light on these novel gifts, and he suddenly decided to consult Mr. Maydig immediately after the service. So soon as that was determined, he found himself wondering why he had not done so before.

Mr. Maydig, a lean, excitable man with quite remarkably long wrists and neck, was gratified at a request for a private conversation from a young man whose carelessness in religious matters was a subject for general remark in the town. After a few necessary delays, he conducted him to the study of the Manse, which was contiguous to the chapel, seated him comfortably, and, standing in front of a cheerful fire—his legs threw a Rhodian arch of shadow on the opposite wall—requested Mr. Fotheringay to state his business.

At first Mr. Fotheringay was a little abashed, and found some difficulty in opening the matter. "You will scarcely believe me, Mr. Maydig, I am afraid"—and so forth for some time. He tried a question at last, and asked Mr. Maydig his opinion of miracles.

Mr. Maydig was still saying "Well" in an extremely judicial tone, when Mr. Fotheringay interrupted again: "You don't believe, I suppose, that some common sort of person—like myself, for instance—as it might be sitting here now, might have some sort of twist inside him that made him able to do things by his will."

"It's possible," said Mr. Maydig. "Something of the sort, perhaps, is possible."

"If I might make free with something here, I think I might show you by a sort of experiment," said Mr. Fotheringay. "Now, take that tobacco-jar on the table, for instance. What I want to know is whether what I am going to do with it is a miracle or not. Just half a minute, Mr. Maydig, please."

He knitted his brows, pointed to the tobacco-jar and said: "Be a bowl of vi'lets."

The tobacco-jar did as it was ordered.

Mr. Maydig started violently at the change, and stood looking from the thaumaturgist to the bowl of flowers. He said nothing. Presently he ventured to lean over the table and smell the violets; they were fresh-picked and very fine ones. Then he stared at Mr. Fotheringay again.

"How did you do that?" he asked.

Mr. Fotheringay pulled his moustache. "Just told it—and there you are. Is that a miracle, or is it black art, or what is it? And what do you think's the matter with me? That's what I want to ask."

"It's a most extraordinary occurrence."

"And this day last week I knew no more that I could do things like that than you did. It came quite sudden. It's something odd about my will, I suppose, and that's as far as I can see."

"Is *that*—the only thing. Could you do other things besides that?"

"Lord, yes!" said Mr. Fotheringay. "Just anything." He thought, and suddenly recalled a conjuring entertainment he had seen. "Here!" He pointed. "Change into a bowl of fish—no, not that—change into a glass bowl full of water with goldfish swimming in it. That's better! You see that, Mr. Maydig?"

"It's astonishing. It's incredible. You are either a most extraordinary . . . But no—"

"I could change it into anything," said Mr. Fotheringay. "Just anything. Here! be a pigeon, will you?"

In another moment a blue pigeon was fluttering round the room and making Mr. Maydig duck every time it came near him. "Stop there, will you," said

Mr. Fotheringay; and the pigeon hung motionless in the air. "I could change it back to a bowl of flowers," he said, and after replacing the pigeon on the table worked that miracle. "I expect you will want your pipe in a bit," he said, and restored the tobacco-jar.

Mr. Maydig had followed all these later changes in a sort of ejaculatory silence. He stared at Mr. Fotheringay and, in a very gingerly manner, picked up the tobacco-jar, examined it, replaced it on the table. "*Well!*" was the only expression of his feelings.

"Now, after that it's easier to explain what I came about," said Mr. Fotheringay; and proceeded to a lengthy and involved narrative of his strange experiences, beginning with the affair of the lamp in the Long Dragon and complicated by persistent allusions to Winch. As he went on, the transient pride Mr. Maydig's consternation had caused passed away; he became the very ordinary Mr. Fotheringay of everyday intercourse again. Mr. Maydig listened intently, the tobacco-jar in his hand, and his bearing changed also with the course of the narrative. Presently, while Mr. Fotheringay was dealing with the miracle of the third egg, the minister interrupted with a fluttering extended hand—

"It is possible," he said. "It is credible. It is amazing, of course, but it reconciles a number of amazing difficulties. The power to work miracles is a gift—a peculiar quality like genius or second sight—hitherto it has come very rarely and to exceptional people. But in this case . . . I have always wondered at the miracles of Mahomet, and at Yogi's miracles, and the miracles of Madame Blavatsky. But, of course! Yes, it is simply a gift! It carries out so beautifully the arguments of that great thinker"—Mr. Maydig's voice sank—"his Grace the Duke of Argyll. Here we plumb some profounder law—deeper than the ordinary laws of nature. Yes—yes. Go on. Go on!"

Mr. Fotheringay proceeded to tell of his misadventure with Winch, and Mr. Maydig, no longer overawed or scared, began to jerk his limbs about and interject astonishment. "It's this what troubled me most," proceeded Mr. Fotheringay; "it's this I'm most mijitly in want of advice for; of course he's at San Francisco—wherever San Francisco may be—but of course it's awkward for both of us, as you'll see, Mr. Maydig. I don't see how he can understand what has happened, and I daresay he's scared and exasperated something tremendous, and trying to get at me. I daresay he keeps on starting off to come here. I send him back, by a miracle, every few hours, when I think of it. And of course, that's a thing he won't be able to understand, and it's bound to annoy him; and, of course, if he takes a ticket every time it will cost him a lot of money. I done the best I could for him, but of course it's difficult for him to put himself in my place. I thought afterwards that his clothes might have got scorched, you know—if Hades is all it's supposed to be—before I shifted him. In that case I suppose they'd have locked him up in San Francisco. Of course I willed him a new suit of clothes on him directly I thought of it. But, you see, I'm already in a deuce of a tangle—"

Mr. Maydig looked serious. "I see you are in a tangle. Yes, it's a difficult position. How you are to end it . . ." He became diffuse and inconclusive.

"However, we'll leave Winch for a little and discuss the larger question. I don't think this is a case of the black art or anything of the sort. I don't think there is any taint of criminality about it at all, Mr. Fotheringay—none whatever, unless you are suppressing material facts. No, it's miracles—pure miracles—miracles, if I may say so, of the very highest class."

He began to pace the hearthrug and gesticulate, while Mr. Fotheringay sat with his arm on the table and his head on his arm, looking worried. "I don't see how I'm to manage about Winch," he said.

"A gift of working miracles—apparently a very powerful gift," said Mr. Maydig, "will find a way about Winch—never fear. My dear Sir, you are a most important man—a man of the most astonishing possibilities. As evidence, for example! And in other ways, the things you may do . . ."

"Yes, *I've* thought of a thing or two," said Mr. Fotheringay. "But—some of the things came a bit twisty. You saw that fish at first? Wrong sort of bowl and wrong sort of fish. And I thought I'd ask someone."

"A proper course," said Mr. Maydig, "a very proper course—altogether the proper course." He stopped and looked at Mr. Fotheringay. "It's practically an unlimited gift. Let us test your powers, for instance. If they really *are* . . . If they really are all they seem to be."

And so, incredible as it may seem, in the study of the little house behind the Congregational Chapel, on the evening of Sunday, Nov. 10, 1896, Mr. Fotheringay, egged on and inspired by Mr. Maydig, began to work miracles. The reader's attention is specially and definitely called to the date. He will object, probably has already objected, that certain points in this story are improbable, that if any things of the sort already described had indeed occurred, they would have been in all the papers a year ago. The details immediately following he will find particularly hard to accept, because among other things they involve the conclusion that he or she, the reader in question, must have been killed in a

violent and unprecedented manner more than a year
ago. Now a miracle is nothing if not improbable, and as
a matter of fact the reader *was* killed in a violent and
unprecedented manner a year ago. In the subsequent
course of this story that will become perfectly clear and
credible, as every right-minded and reasonable reader
will admit. But this is not the place for the end of the
story, being but little beyond the hither side of the middle. And at first the miracles worked by Mr. Fotheringay were timid little miracles—little things with the
cups and parlour fitments, as feeble as the miracles of
Theosophists, and, feeble as they were, they were received with awe by his collaborator. He would have
preferred to settle the Winch business out of hand, but
Mr. Maydig would not let him. But after they had
worked a dozen of these domestic trivialities, their
sense of power grew, their imagination began to show
signs of stimulation, and their ambition enlarged. Their
first larger enterprise was due to hunger and the negli-
gence of Mrs. Minchin, Mr. Maydig's housekeeper.
The meal to which the minister conducted Mr. Fotheringay was certainly ill-laid and uninviting as refresh-
ment for two industrious miracle-workers; but they
were seated, and Mr. Maydig was descanting in sorrow
rather than in anger upon his housekeeper's shortcom-
ings, before it occurred to Mr. Fotheringay that an
opportunity lay before him. "Don't you think, Mr.
Maydig," he said, "if it isn't a liberty, I—"

"My dear Mr. Fotheringay! Of course! No—I didn't
think."

Mr. Fotheringay waved his hand. "What shall we
have?" he said, in a large, inclusive spirit, and, at
Mr. Maydig's order, revised the supper very thoroughly.
"As for me," he said, eyeing Mr. Maydig's selection, "I

am always particularly fond of a tankard of stout and a nice Welsh rarebit, and I'll order that. I ain't much given to Burgundy," and forthwith stout and Welsh rarebit promptly appeared at his command. They sat long at their supper, talking like equals, as Mr. Fotheringay presently perceived, with a glow of surprise and gratification, of all the miracles they would presently do. "And, by the bye, Mr. Maydig," said Mr. Fotheringay, "I might perhaps be able to help you—in a domestic way."

"Don't quite follow," said Mr. Maydig pouring out a glass of miraculous old Burgundy.

Mr. Fotheringay helped himself to a second Welsh rarebit out of vacancy, and took a mouthful. "I was thinking," he said, "I might be able (*chum, chum*) to work (*chum, chum*) a miracle with Mrs. Minchin (*chum, chum*)—make her a better woman."

Mr. Maydig put down the glass and looked doubtful. "She's—She strongly objects to interference, you know, Mr. Fotheringay. And—as a matter of fact—it's well past eleven and she's probably in bed and asleep. Do you think, on the whole—"

Mr. Fotheringay considered these objections. "I don't see that it shouldn't be done in her sleep."

For a time Mr. Maydig opposed the idea, and then he yielded. Mr. Fotheringay issued his orders, and a little less at their ease, perhaps, the two gentlemen proceeded with their repast. Mr. Maydig was enlarging on the changes he might expect in his housekeeper next day, with an optimism that seemed even to Mr. Fotheringay's supper senses a little forced and hectic, when a series of confused noises from upstairs began. Their eyes exchanged interrogations, and Mr. Maydig left the room hastily. Mr. Fotheringay heard him calling up to his housekeeper and then his footsteps going softly up to her.

In a minute or so the minister returned, his step light, his face radiant. "Wonderful!" he said, "and touching! Most touching!"

He began pacing the hearthrug. "A repentance—a most touching repentance—through the crack of the door. Poor woman! A most wonderful change! She had got up. She must have got up at once. She had got up out of her sleep to smash a private bottle of brandy in her box. And to confess it too! . . . But this gives us—it opens—a most amazing vista of possibilities. If we can work this miraculous change in *her* . . ."

"The thing's unlimited seemingly," said Mr. Fotheringay. "And about Mr. Winch—"

"Altogether unlimited." And from the hearthrug Mr. Maydig, waving the Winch difficulty aside, unfolded a series of wonderful proposals—proposals he invented as he went along.

Now what those proposals were does not concern the essentials of this story. Suffice it that they were designed in a spirit of infinite benevolence, the sort of benevolence that used to be called post-prandial. Suffice it, too, that the problem of Winch remained unsolved. Nor is it necessary to describe how far that series got to its fulfilment. There were astonishing changes. The small hours found Mr. Maydig and Mr. Fotheringay career-ing across the chilly market-square under the still moon, in a sort of ecstasy of thaumaturgy, Mr. Maydig all flap and gesture, Mr. Fotheringay short and bris-tling, and no longer abashed at his greatness. They had reformed every drunkard in the Parliamentary division, changed all the beer and alcohol to water (Mr. Maydig had overruled Mr. Fotheringay on this point); they had, further, greatly improved the railway communication of the place, drained Flinder's swamp, improved the soil of One Tree Hill, and cured the Vicar's wart. And they were going to see what could be done with the injured pier at South Bridge. "The place," gasped Mr. Maydig, "won't be the same place to-morrow. How surprised and thankful everyone will be!" And just at that moment the church clock struck three.

"I say," said Mr. Fotheringay, "that's three o'clock! I must be getting back. I've got to be at business by eight. And besides, Mrs. Wimms—"

"We're only beginning," said Mr. Maydig, full of the sweetness of unlimited power. "We're only beginning. Think of all the good we're doing. When people wake—"

"But—," said Mr. Fotheringay.

Mr. Maydig gripped his arm suddenly. His eyes were bright and wild. "My dear chap," he said, "there's no hurry. Look"—he pointed to the moon at the zenith—"Joshua!"

"Joshua?" said Mr. Fotheringay.

"Joshua," said Mr. Maydig. "Why not? Stop it."

Mr. Fotheringay looked at the moon.

"That's a bit tall," he said after a pause.

"Why not?" said Mr. Maydig. "Of course it doesn't stop. You stop the rotation of the earth, you know. Time stops. It isn't as if we were doing harm."

"H'm!" said Mr. Fotheringay. "Well." He sighed. "I'll try. Here—"

He buttoned up his jacket and addressed himself to the habitable globe, with as good an assumption of confidence as lay in his power. "Jest stop rotating, will you," said Mr. Fotheringay.

Incontinently he was flying head over heels through the air at the rate of dozens of miles a minute. In spite of the innumerable circles he was describing per second, he thought; for thought is wonderful—sometimes as sluggish as flowing pitch, sometimes as instantaneous as light. He thought in a second, and willed. "Let me come down safe and sound. Whatever else happens, let me down safe and sound."

He willed it only just in time, for his clothes, heated by his rapid flight through the air, were already beginning to singe. He came down with a forcible, but by no means injurious bump in what appeared to be a mound of fresh-turned earth. A large mass of metal and masonry, extraordinarily like the clock-tower in the middle of the market-square, hit the earth near him, ricocheted over him, and flew into stonework, bricks, and masonry, like a bursting bomb. A hurtling cow hit one of the larger blocks and smashed like an egg. There was a crash that made all the most violent crashes of his past life seem like the sound of falling dust, and this was followed by a descending series of lesser crashes. A vast wind roared throughout earth and heaven, so that he could scarcely lift his head to look. For a while he was too breathless and astonished even to see where he was or what had happened. And his first movement was to feel his head and reassure himself that his streaming hair was still his own.

"Lord!" gasped Mr. Fotheringay, scarce able to speak for the gale, "I've had a squeak! What's gone wrong? Storms and thunder. And only a minute ago a fine night. It's Maydig set me on to this sort of thing. *What* a wind! If I go on fooling in this way I'm bound to have a thundering accident! . . .

"Where's Maydig?

"What a confounded mess everything's in!"

He looked about him so far as his flapping jacket

would permit. The appearance of things was really extremely strange. "The sky's all right anyhow," said Mr. Fotheringay. "And that's about all that is all right. And even there it looks like a terrific gale coming up. But there's the moon overhead. Just as it was just now. Bright as midday. But as for the rest—Where's the village? Where's—where's anything? And what on earth set this wind a-blowing? *I* didn't order no wind."

Mr. Fotheringay struggled to get to his feet in vain, and after one failure, remained on all fours, holding on. He surveyed the moonlit world to leeward, with the tails of his jacket streaming over his head. "There's something seriously wrong," said Mr. Fotheringay. "And what it is—goodness knows."

Far and wide nothing was visible in the white glare through the haze of dust that drove before a screaming gale but tumbled masses of earth and heaps of inchoate ruins, no trees, no houses, no familiar shapes, only a wilderness of disorder vanishing at last into the darkness beneath the whirling columns and streamers, the lightnings and thunderings of a swiftly rising storm. Near him in the livid glare was something that might once have been an elm-tree, a smashed mass of splinters, shivered from boughs to base, and further a twisted mass of iron girders—only too evidently the viaduct—rose out of the piled confusion.

You see, when Mr. Fotheringay had arrested the rotation of the solid globe, he had made no stipulation concerning the trifling movables upon its surface. And the earth spins so fast that the surface at its equator is travelling at rather more than a thousand miles an hour, and in these latitudes at more than half that pace. So that the village, and Mr. Maydig, and Mr. Fotheringay, and everybody and everything had been jerked violently forward at about nine miles per second—that is to say, much more violently than if they had been fired out of a cannon. And every human being, every living creature, every house, and every tree—all the world as we know it—had been so jerked and smashed and utterly destroyed. That was all.

These things Mr. Fotheringay did not, of course, fully appreciate. But he perceived that his miracle had miscarried, and with that a great disgust of miracles came upon him. He was in darkness now, for the clouds had swept together and blotted out his momentary glimpse of the moon, and the air was full of fitful struggling tortured wraiths of hail. A great roaring of wind and waters filled earth and sky, and, peering under his hand through the dust and sleet to windward, he saw by the play of the lightnings a vast wall of water pouring towards him.

"Maydig!" screamed Mr. Fotheringay's feeble voice amid the elemental uproar. "Here!—Maydig!

"Stop!" cried Mr. Fotheringay to the advancing water. "Oh, for goodness' sake, stop!

"Just a moment," said Mr. Fotheringay to the lightnings and thunder. "Stop jest a moment while I collect my thoughts . . . And now what shall I do?" he said. "What *shall* I do? Lord! I wish Maydig was about.

"I know," said Mr. Fotheringay. "And for goodness' sake let's have it right *this* time."

He remained on all fours, leaning against the wind, very intent to have everything right.

"Ah!" he said. "Let nothing what I'm going to order happen until I say 'Off!' . . . Lord! I wish I'd thought of that before!"

He lifted his little voice against the whirlwind, shouting louder and louder in the vain desire to hear himself speak. "Now then!—here goes! Mind about that what I said just now. In the first place, when all I've got to say is done, let me lose my miraculous power, let my will become just like anybody else's will, and all these dangerous miracles be stopped. I don't like them. I'd rather I didn't work 'em. Ever so much. That's the first thing. And the second is—let me be back just before the miracles begin; let everything be just as it was before that blessed lamp turned up. It's a big job, but it's the last. Have you got it? No more miracles, everything as it was—me back in the Long Dragon just before I drank my half-pint. That's it! Yes."

He dug his fingers into the mould, closed his eyes, and said "Off!"

Everything became perfectly still. He perceived that he was standing erect.

"So *you* say," said a voice.

He opened his eyes. He was in the bar of the Long Dragon, arguing about miracles with Toddy Beamish. He had a vague sense of some great thing forgotten that instantaneously passed. You see that, except for the loss of his miraculous powers, everything was back as it had been, his mind and memory therefore were now just as they had been at the time when this story began. So that he knew absolutely nothing of all that is told here, knows nothing of all that is told here to this day. And among other things, of course, he still did not believe in miracles.

"I tell you that miracles, properly speaking, can't possibly happen," he said, "whatever you like to hold. And I'm prepared to prove it up to the hilt."

"That's what *you* think," said Toddy Beamish, and "Prove it if you can."

"Looky here, Mr. Beamish," said Mr. Fotheringay. "Let us clearly understand what a miracle is. It's something contrariwise to the course of nature done by power of Will . . ."

WILLA CATHER

The Burglar's Christmas

Two very shabby looking young men stood at the corner of Prairie avenue and Eightieth street, looking despondently at the carriages that whirled by. It was Christmas Eve, and the streets were full of vehicles; florists' wagons, grocers' carts and carriages. The streets were in that half-liquid, half-congealed condition peculiar to the streets of Chicago at that season of the year. The swift wheels that spun by sometimes threw the slush of mud and snow over the two young men who were talking on the corner.

"Well," remarked the elder of the two, "I guess we are at our rope's end, sure enough. How do you feel?"

"Pretty shaky. The wind's sharp to-night. If I had had anything to eat I mightn't mind it so much. There is simply no show. I'm sick of the whole business. Looks like there's nothing for it but the lake."

"O, nonsense, I thought you had more grit. Got anything left you can hoc?"

"Nothing but my beard, and I am afraid they wouldn't find it worth a pawn ticket," said the younger man ruefully, rubbing the week's growth of stubble on his face.

"Got any folks anywhere? Now's your time to strike 'em if you have."

"Never mind if I have, they're out of the question."

"Well, you'll be out of it before many hours if you don't make a move of some sort. A man's got to eat.

See here, I am going down to Longtin's saloon. I used to play the banjo in there with a couple of guys, and I'll bone him for some of his free lunch stuff. You'd better come along, perhaps they'll fill an order for two."

"How far down is it?"

"Well, it's clear down town, of course, way down on Michigan avenue."

"Thanks, I guess I'll loaf around here. I don't feel equal to the walk, and the cars—well, the cars are crowded." His features drew themselves into what might have been a smile under happier circumstances.

"No, you never did like street cars, you're too aristocratic. See here, Crawford, I don't like leaving you here. You ain't good company for yourself to-night."

"Crawford? O, yes, that's the last one. There have been so many I forget them."

"Have you got a real name, anyway?"

"O, yes, but it's one of the ones I've forgotten. Don't you worry about me. You go along and get your free lunch. I think I had a row in Longtin's place once. I'd better not show myself there again." As he spoke the young man nodded and turned slowly up the avenue.

He was miserable enough to want to be quite alone. Even the crowd that jostled by him annoyed him. He wanted to think about himself. He had avoided this final reckoning with himself for a year now. He had laughed it off and drunk it off. But now, when all those artificial devices which are employed to turn our thoughts into other channels and shield us from ourselves had failed him, it must come. Hunger is a powerful incentive to introspection.

It is a tragic hour, that hour when we are finally driven to reckon with ourselves, when every avenue of mental distraction has been cut off and our own life and all its ineffaceable failures closes about us like the walls of that old torture chamber of the Inquisition. To-night, as this man stood stranded in the streets of the city, his hour came. It was not the first time he had been hungry and desperate and alone. But always before there had been some outlook, some chance ahead, some pleasure yet untasted that seemed worth the effort, some face that he fancied was, or would be, dear. But it was not so to-night. The unyielding conviction was upon him that he had failed in everything, had outlived everything. It had been near him for a long time, that Pale Spectre. He had caught its shadow at the bottom of his glass many a time, at the head of his bed when he was sleepless at night, in the twilight shadows when some great sunset broke upon him. It had made life hateful to him when he awoke in the morning before now. But now it settled slowly over him, like night, the endless Northern nights that bid the sun a long farewell. It rose up before him like granite. From this brilliant city with its glad bustle of Yule-tide he was shut off as completely as though he were a creature of another species. His days seemed numbered and done, sealed over like the little coral cells at the bottom of the sea. Involuntarily he drew that cold air through his lungs slowly, as though he were tasting it for the last time.

Yet he was but four and twenty, this man—he looked even younger—and he had a father some place down East who had been very proud of him once. Well, he had taken his life into his own hands, and this was what he had made of it. That was all there was to be said. He could remember the hopeful things they used to say about him at college in the old days, before he had cut away and begun to live by his wits, and he found courage to smile at them now. They had read him wrongly. He knew now that he never had the essentials of success, only the superficial agility that is often mistaken for it. He was tow without the tinder, and he had burnt himself out at other people's fires. He had helped other people to make it win, but he himself—he had never touched an enterprise that had not failed eventually. Or, if it survived his connection with it, it left him behind.

His last venture had been with some ten-cent specialty company, a little lower than all the others, that had gone to pieces in Buffalo, and he had worked his way to Chicago by boat. When the boat made up its crew for the outward voyage, he was dispensed with as usual. He was used to that. The reason for it? O, there are so many reasons for failure! His was a very common one.

As he stood there in the wet under the street light he drew up his reckoning with the world and decided that it had treated him as well as he deserved. He had overdrawn his account once too often. There had been a day when he thought otherwise; when he had said he was unjustly handled, that his failure was merely the lack of proper adjustment between himself and other men, that some day he would be recognized and it would all come right. But he knew better than that now, and he was still man enough to bear no grudge against anyone—man or woman.

To-night was his birthday, too. There seemed something particularly amusing in that. He turned up a limp little coat collar to try to keep a little of the wet chill from his throat, and instinctively began to remember all the birthday parties he used to have. He was so cold and empty that his mind seemed unable to grapple with any serious question. He kept thinking about ginger bread and frosted cakes like a child. He could remember the splendid birthday parties his mother used to give him, when all the other little boys in the block came in their Sunday clothes and creaking shoes, with their ears still red from their mother's towel, and the pink and white birthday cake, and the stuffed olives and all the dishes of which he had been particularly fond, and how he would eat and eat and then go to bed and dream of Santa Claus. And in the morning he would awaken and eat again, until by night the family doctor arrived with his castor oil, and poor William used to dolefully say that it was altogether too much to have your birthday and Christmas all at once. He could remember, too, the royal birthday suppers he had given at college, and the stag dinners, and the toasts, and the music, and the good fellows who had wished him happiness and really meant what they said.

And since then there were other birthday suppers that he could not remember so clearly; the memory of them was heavy and flat, like cigarette smoke that has been shut in a room all night, like champagne that has been a day opened, a song that has been too often sung, an acute sensation that has been overstrained. They seemed tawdry and garish, discordant to him now. He rather wished he could forget them altogether.

Whichever way his mind now turned there was one thought that it could not escape, and that was the idea of food. He caught the scent of a cigar suddenly, and felt a sharp pain in the pit of his abdomen and a sudden moisture in his mouth. His cold hands clenched angrily, and for a moment he felt that bitter hatred of wealth, of ease, of everything that is well-fed and well-housed that is common to starving men. At any rate he had a right to eat! He had demanded great things from the world once: fame and wealth and admiration. Now it was simply bread—and he would have it! He looked about him quickly and felt the blood begin to stir in his veins. In all his straits he had never stolen anything, his tastes were above it. But to-night there would be no to-morrow. He was amused at the way in which the idea excited him. Was it possible there was yet one more experience that would distract him, one thing that had power to excite his jaded interest? Good! he had failed at everything else, now he would see what his chances would be as a common thief. It would be amusing to watch the beautiful consistency of his destiny work itself out even in that role. It would be interesting to add another study to his gallery of futile attempts, and then label them all: "the failure as a journalist," "the failure as a lecturer," "the failure as a business man," "the failure as a thief," and so on, like the titles under the pictures of the Dance of Death. It was time that Childe Roland came to the dark tower.

A girl hastened by him with her arms full of packages. She walked quickly and nervously, keeping well within the shadow, as if she were not accustomed to carrying bundles and did not care to meet any of her friends. As she crossed the muddy street, she made an effort to lift her skirt a little, and as she did so one of the packages slipped unnoticed from beneath her arm. He caught it up and overtook her. "Excuse me, but I think you dropped something."

She started, "O, yes, thank you, I would rather have lost anything than that."

The young man turned angrily upon himself. The package must have contained something of value. Why had he not kept it? Was this the sort of thief he would make? He ground his teeth together. There is nothing more maddening than to have morally consented to crime and then lack the nerve force to carry it out.

A carriage drove up to the house before which he stood. Several richly dressed women alighted and went in. It was a new house, and must have been built since he was in Chicago last. The front door was open and he could see down the hall-way and up the stair case. The servant had left the door and gone with the guests. The first floor was brilliantly lighted, but the windows upstairs were dark. It looked very easy, just to slip up-stairs to the darkened chambers where the jewels and trinkets of the fashionable occupants were kept.

Still burning with impatience against himself he entered quickly. Instinctively he removed his mud-stained hat as he passed quickly and quietly up the stair case. It struck him as being a rather superfluous courtesy in a burglar, but he had done it before he had thought. His way was clear enough, he met no one on the stairway or in the upper hall. The gas was lit in the upper hall. He passed the first chamber door through sheer cowardice. The second he entered quickly, thinking of something else lest his courage should fail him, and closed the door behind him. The light from the hall shone into the room through the transom. The apartment was furnished richly enough to justify his expectations. He went at once to the dressing case. A number of rings and small trinkets lay in a silver tray. These he put hastily in his pocket. He opened the upper drawer and found, as he expected, several leather cases. In the first he opened was a lady's watch, in the second a pair of old-fashioned bracelets; he seemed to dimly remember having seen bracelets like them before, somewhere. The third case was heavier, the spring was much worn, and it opened easily. It held a cup of some kind. He held it up to the light and then his strained nerves gave way and he uttered a sharp exclamation. It was the silver mug he used to drink from when he was a little boy.

The door opened, and a woman stood in the doorway facing him. She was a tall woman, with white hair, in evening dress. The light from the hall streamed in upon him, but she was not afraid. She stood looking at him a moment, then she threw out her hand and went quickly toward him.

"Willie, Willie! Is it you!"

He struggled to loose her arms from him, to keep her lips from his cheek. "Mother—you must not! You do not understand! O, my God, this is worst of all!" Hunger, weakness, cold, shame, all came back to him, and shook his self-control completely. Physically he was too weak to stand a shock like this. Why could it not have been an ordinary discovery, arrest, the station house and all the rest of it. Anything but this! A hard dry sob broke from him. Again he strove to disengage himself.

"Who is it says I shall not kiss my son? O, my boy, we have waited so long for this! You have been so long in coming, even I almost gave you up."

Her lips upon his cheek burnt him like fire. He put his hand to his throat, and spoke thickly and incoherently: "You do not understand. I did not know you were here. I came here to rob—it is the first time—I swear it—but I am a common thief. My pockets are full of your jewels now. Can't you hear me? I am a common thief!"

"Hush, my boy, those are ugly words. How could you rob your own house? How could you take what is your own? They are all yours, my son, as wholly yours as my great love—and you can't doubt that, Will, do you?"

That soft voice, the warmth and fragrance of her person stole through his chill, empty veins like a gentle stimulant. He felt as though all his strength were leaving him and even consciousness. He held fast to her and bowed his head on her strong shoulder, and groaned aloud.

"O, mother, life is hard, hard!"

She said nothing, but held him closer. And O, the strength of those white arms that held him! O, the assurance of safety in that warm bosom that rose and fell under his cheek! For a moment they stood so, silently. Then they heard a heavy step upon the stair. She led him to a chair and went out and closed the door. At the top of the staircase she met a tall, broad-shouldered man, with iron grey hair, and a face alert and stern. Her eyes were shining and her cheeks on fire, her whole face was one expression of intense determination.

"James, it is William in there, come home. You must keep him at any cost. If he goes this time, I go with him. O, James, be easy with him, he has suffered so." She broke from a command to an entreaty, and laid her hand on his shoulder. He looked questioningly at her a moment, then went in the room and quietly shut the door.

She stood leaning against the wall, clasping her temples with her hands and listening to the low indistinct sound of the voices within. Her own lips moved silently. She waited a long time, scarcely breathing. At last the door opened, and her husband came out. He stopped to say in a shaken voice,

"You go to him now, he will stay. I will go to my room. I will see him again in the morning."

She put her arm about his neck, "O, James, I thank you, I thank you! This is the night he came so long ago, you remember? I gave him to you then, and now you give him back to me!"

"Don't, Helen," he muttered. "He is my son, I have never forgotten that. I failed with him. I don't like to fail, it cuts my pride. Take him and make a man of him." He passed on down the hall.

She flew into the room where the young man sat with his head bowed upon his knee. She dropped upon her knees beside him. Ah, it was so good to him to feel those arms again!

"He is so glad, Willie, so glad! He may not show it, but he is as happy as I. He never was demonstrative with either of us, you know."

"O, my God, he was good enough," groaned the man. "I told him everything, and he was good enough. I don't see how either of you can look at me, speak to me, touch me." He shivered under her clasp again as when she had first touched him, and tried weakly to throw her off.

But she whispered softly,

"This is my right, my son."

Presently, when he was calmer, she rose. "Now, come with me into the library, and I will have your dinner brought there."

As they went down stairs she remarked apologetically, "I will not call Ellen to-night; she has a number of guests to attend to. She is a big girl now, you know, and came out last winter. Besides, I want you all to myself to-night."

When the dinner came, and it came very soon, he fell upon it savagely. As he ate she told him all that had transpired during the years of his absence, and how his father's business had brought them there. "I was glad when we came. I thought you would drift West. I seemed a good deal nearer to you here."

There was a gentle unobtrusive sadness in her tone that was too soft for a reproach.

"Have you everything you want? It is a comfort to see you eat."

He smiled grimly, "It is certainly a comfort to me. I have not indulged in this frivolous habit for some thirty-five hours."

She caught his hand and pressed it sharply, uttering a quick remonstrance.

"Don't say that! I know, but I can't hear you say it,—it's too terrible! My boy, food has choked me many a time when I have thought of the possibility of that. Now take the old lounging chair by the fire, and if you are too tired to talk, we will just sit and rest together."

He sank into the depths of the big leather chair with the lion's heads on the arms, where he had sat so often in the days when his feet did not touch the floor and he was half afraid of the grim monsters cut in the polished wood. That chair seemed to speak to him of things long forgotten. It was like the touch of an old familiar friend. He felt a sudden yearning tenderness for the happy little boy who had sat there and dreamed of the big world so long ago. Alas, he had been dead many a summer, that little boy!

He sat looking up at the magnificent woman beside him. He had almost forgotten how handsome she was; how lustrous and sad were the eyes that were set under that serene brow, how impetuous and wayward the mouth even now, how superb the white throat and shoulders! Ah, the wit and grace and fineness of this woman! He remembered how proud he had been of her as a boy when she came to see him at school. Then in the deep red coals of the grate he saw the faces of other women who had come since then into his vexed, disordered life. Laughing faces, with eyes artificially bright, eyes without depth or meaning, features without the stamp of high sensibilities. And he had left this face for such as those!

He sighed restlessly and laid his hand on hers. There seemed refuge and protection in the touch of her, as in the old days when he was afraid of the dark. He had been in the dark so long now, his confidence was so thoroughly shaken, and he was bitterly afraid of the night and of himself.

"Ah, mother, you make other things seem so false. You must feel that I owe you an explanation, but I can't make any, even to myself. Ah, but we make poor exchanges in life. I can't make out the riddle of it all. Yet there are things I ought to tell you before I accept your confidence like this."

"I'd rather you wouldn't, Will. Listen: Between you and me there can be no secrets. We are more alike than other people. Dear boy, I know all about it. I am a woman, and circumstances were different with me, but we are of one blood. I have lived all your life before you. You have never had an impulse that I have not known, you have never touched a brink that my feet have not trod. This is your birthday night. Twenty-four years ago I foresaw all this. I was a young woman then and I had hot battles of my own, and I felt your likeness to me. You were not like other babies. From the hour you were born you were restless and discontented, as I had been before you. You used to brace your strong little limbs against mine and try to throw me off as you did tonight. To-night you have come back to me, just as you always did after you ran away to swim in the river that was forbidden you, the river you loved because it was forbidden. You are tired and sleepy, just as you used to be then, only a little older and a little paler and a little more foolish. I never asked you where you had been then, nor will I now. You have come back to me, that's all in all to me. I know your every possibility and limitation, as a composer knows his instrument."

He found no answer that was worthy to give to talk like this. He had not found life easy since he had lived by his wits. He had come to know poverty at close quarters. He had known what it was to be gay with an empty pocket, to wear violets in his button hole when he had not breakfasted, and all the hateful shams of the poverty of idleness. He had been a reporter on a big metropolitan daily, where men grind out their brains on paper until they have not one idea left—and still grind on. He had worked in a real estate office, where ignorant men were swindled. He had sung in a comic opera chorus and played *Harris* in an Uncle Tom's Cabin Company, and edited a Socialist weekly. He had been dogged by debt and hunger and grinding poverty, until to sit here by a warm fire without concern as to how it would be paid for seemed unnatural.

He looked up at her questioningly. "I wonder if you know how much you pardon?"

"O, my poor boy, much or little, what does it matter? Have you wandered so far and paid such a bitter price for knowledge and not yet learned that love has nothing to do with pardon or forgiveness, that it only loves, and loves—and loves? They have not taught you well, the women of your world." She leaned over and kissed him, as no woman had kissed him since he left her.

He drew a long sigh of rich content. The old life, with all its bitterness and useless antagonism and flimsy sophistries, its brief delights that were always tinged with fear and distrust and unfaith, that whole miserable, futile, swindled world of Bohemia seemed immeasurably distant and far away, like a dream that is over and done. And as the chimes rang joyfully outside and sleep pressed heavily upon his eyelids, he wondered dimly if the Author of this sad little riddle of ours were not able to solve it after all, and if the Potter would not finally mete out his all comprehensive justice, such as none but he could have, to his Things of Clay, which are made in his own patterns, weak or strong, for his own ends; and if some day we will not awaken and find that all evil is a dream, a mental distortion that will pass when the dawn shall break.

ANTON CHEKHOV

A Story Without a Title

In the fifth century, just as now, the sun rose every
morning and every evening retired to rest. In the morning, when the first rays kissed the dew, the earth revived, the air was filled with the sounds of rapture and
hope; while in the evening the same earth subsided into
silence and plunged into gloomy darkness. One day was
like another, one night like another. From time to time
a storm-cloud raced up and there was the angry rumble
of thunder, or a negligent star fell out of the sky, or a
pale monk ran to tell the brotherhood that not far from
the monastery he had seen a tiger—and that was all,
and then each day was like the next.

The monks worked and prayed, and their Father
Superior played on the organ, made Latin verses, and
wrote music. The wonderful old man possessed an
extraordinary gift. He played on the organ with such art
that even the oldest monks, whose hearing had grown
somewhat dull towards the end of their lives, could not
restrain their tears when the sounds of the organ floated
from his cell. When he spoke of anything, even of the
most ordinary things—for instance of the trees, of the
wild beasts, or of the sea—they could not listen to him
without a smile or tears, and it seemed that the same
chords vibrated in his soul as in the organ. If he were
moved to anger or abandoned himself to intense joy, or
began speaking of something terrible or grand, then a
passionate inspiration took possession of him, tears

came into his flashing eyes, his face flushed, and his voice thundered, and as the monks listened to him they felt that their souls were spell-bound by his inspiration; at such marvellous, splendid moments his power over them was boundless, and if he had bidden his elders fling themselves into the sea, they would all, every one of them, have hastened to carry out his wishes.

His music, his voice, his poetry in which he glorified God, the heavens and the earth, were a continual source of joy to the monks. It sometimes happened that through the monotony of their lives they grew weary of the trees, the flowers, the spring, the autumn, their ears were tired of the sound of the sea, and the song of the birds seemed tedious to them, but the talents of their Father Superior were as necessary to them as their daily bread.

Dozens of years passed by, and every day was like every other day, every night was like every other night. Except the birds and the wild beasts, not one soul appeared near the monastery. The nearest human habitation was far away, and to reach it from the monastery, or to reach the monastery from it, meant a journey of over seventy miles across the desert. Only men who despised life, who had renounced it, and who came to the monastery as to the grave, ventured to cross the desert.

What was the amazement of the monks, therefore, when one night there knocked at their gate a man who turned out to be from the town, and the most ordinary sinner who loved life. Before saying his prayers and asking for the Father Superior's blessing, this man asked for wine and food. To the question how he had come from the town into the desert, he answered by a long story of hunting; he had gone out hunting, had drunk too much, and lost his way. To the suggestion that he should enter the monastery and save his soul, he replied with a smile: "I am not a fit companion for you!"

When he had eaten and drunk he looked at the monks who were serving him, shook his head reproachfully, and said:

"You don't do anything, you monks. You are good for nothing but eating and drinking. Is that the way to save one's soul? Only think, while you sit here in peace, eat and drink and dream of beatitude, your neighbours are perishing and going to hell. You should see what is going on in the town! Some are dying of hunger, others, not knowing what to do with their gold, sink into profligacy and perish like flies stuck in honey. There is no faith, no truth in men. Whose task is it to save them? Whose work is it to preach to them? It is not for me, drunk from morning till night as I am. Can a meek spirit, a loving heart, and faith in God have been given you for you to sit here within four walls doing nothing?"

The townsman's drunken words were insolent and unseemly, but they had a strange effect upon the Father Superior. The old man exchanged glances with his monks, turned pale, and said:

"My brothers, he speaks the truth, you know. Indeed, poor people in their weakness and lack of understanding are perishing in vice and infidelity, while we do not move, as though it did not concern us. Why should I not go and remind them of the Christ whom they have forgotten?"

The townsman's words had carried the old man away. The next day he took his staff, said farewell to the brotherhood, and set off for the town. And the monks were left without music, and without his speeches and verses.

They spent a month drearily, then a second, but the old man did not come back. At last after three months had passed the familiar tap of his staff was heard. The monks flew to meet him and showered questions upon him, but instead of being delighted to see them he wept bitterly and did not utter a word. The monks noticed that he looked greatly aged and had grown thinner; his face looked exhausted and wore an expression of profound sadness, and when he wept he had the air of a man who has been outraged.

The monks fell to weeping too, and began with sympathy asking him why he was weeping, why his face was so gloomy, but he locked himself in his cell without uttering a word. For seven days he sat in his cell, eating and drinking nothing, weeping and not playing on his organ. To knocking at his door and to the entreaties of the monks to come out and share his grief with them he replied with unbroken silence.

At last he came out. Gathering all the monks around him, with a tear-stained face and with an expression of grief and indignation, he began telling them of what had befallen him during those three months. His voice was calm and his eyes were smiling while he described his journey from the monastery to the town. On the road, he told them, the birds sang to him, the brooks gurgled, and sweet youthful hopes agitated his soul; he marched on and felt like a soldier going to battle and confident of victory; he walked on dreaming, and composed poems and hymns, and reached the end of his journey without noticing it.

But his voice quivered, his eyes flashed, and he was full of wrath when he came to speak of the town and of the men in it. Never in his life had he seen or even dared to imagine what he met with when he went into the town. Only then for the first time in his life, in his old age, he saw and understood how powerful was the devil, how fair was evil and how weak and faint-hearted and worthless were men. By an unhappy chance the first dwelling he entered was the abode of vice. Some fifty men in possession of much money were eating and drinking wine beyond measure. Intoxicated by the wine, they sang songs and boldly uttered terrible, revolting words such as a God-fearing man could not bring himself to pronounce; boundlessly free, self-confident, and happy, they feared neither God nor the devil, nor death, but said and did what they liked, and went whither their lust led them. And the wine, clear as amber, flecked with sparks of gold, must have been irresistibly sweet and fragrant, for each man who drank it smiled blissfully and wanted to drink more.

To the smile of man it responded with a smile and sparkled joyfully when they drank it, as though it knew the devilish charm it kept hidden in its sweetness.

The old man, growing more and more incensed and weeping with wrath, went on to describe what he had seen. On a table in the midst of the revellers, he said, stood a sinful, half-naked woman. It was hard to imagine or to find in nature anything more lovely and fascinating. This reptile, young, longhaired, dark-skinned, with black eyes and full lips, shameless and insolent, showed her snow-white teeth and smiled as though to say: "Look how shameless, how beautiful I am." Silk and brocade fell in lovely folds from her shoulders, but her beauty would not hide itself under her clothes, but eagerly thrust itself through the folds, like the young grass through the ground in spring. The shameless woman drank wine, sang songs, and abandoned herself to anyone who wanted her.

Then the old man, wrathfully brandishing his arms, described the horse-races, the bull-fights, the theatres, the artists' studios where they painted naked women or moulded them of clay. He spoke with inspiration, with sonorous beauty, as though he were playing on unseen chords, while the monks, petrified, greedily drank in his words and gasped with rapture . . .

After describing all the charms of the devil, the beauty of evil, and the fascinating grace of the dreadful female form, the old man cursed the devil, turned and shut himself up in his cell . . .

When he came out of his cell in the morning there was not a monk left in the monastery; they had all fled to the town.

A Modern Cinderella; or, The Little Old Shoe

HOW IT WAS LOST

Among green New England hills stood an ancient house, many-gabled, mossy-roofed, and quaintly built, but picturesque and pleasant to the eye; for a brook ran babbling through the orchard that encompassed it about, a garden-plat stretched upward to the whispering birches on the slope, and patriarchal elms stood sentinel upon the lawn, as they had stood almost a century ago, when the Revolution rolled that way and found them young.

One summer morning, when the air was full of country sounds, of mowers in the meadow, black-birds by the brook, and the low of kine upon the hill-side, the old house wore its cheeriest aspect, and a certain humble history began.

"Nan!"

"Yes, Di."

And a head, brown-locked, blue-eyed, soft-featured, looked in at the open door in answer to the call.

"Just bring me the third volume of 'Wilhelm Meister,' there's a dear. It's hardly worthwhile to rouse such a restless ghost as I, when I'm once fairly laid."

As she spoke, Di pulled up her black braids, thumped the pillow of the couch where she was lying, and with eager eyes went down the last page of her book.

"Nan!"

"Yes, Laura," replied the girl, coming back with the third volume for the literary cormorant, who took it with a nod, still too content upon the "Confessions of a Fair Saint" to remember the failings of a certain plain sinner.

"Don't forget the Italian cream for dinner. I depend upon it; for it's the only thing fit for me this hot weather."

And Laura, the cool blonde, disposed the folds of her white gown more gracefully about her, and touched up the eyebrow of the Minerva she was drawing.

"Little daughter!"

"Yes, father."

"Let me have plenty of clean collars in my bag, for I must go at once; and some of you bring me a glass of cider in about an hour;—I shall be in the lower garden."

The old man went away into his imaginary paradise, and Nan into that domestic purgatory on a summer day,—the kitchen. There were vines about the windows, sunshine on the floor, and order everywhere; but it was haunted by a cooking-stove, that family altar whence such varied incense rises to appease the appetite of household gods, before which such dire incantations are pronounced to ease the wrath and woe of the priestess of the fire, and about which often linger saddest memories of wasted temper, time, and toil.

Nan was tired, having risen with the birds,—hurried, having many cares those happy little housewives never know,—and disappointed in a hope that hourly "dwindled, peaked, and pined." She was too young to make the anxious lines upon her forehead seem at home there, too patient to be burdened with the labour others should have shared, too light of heart to be pent up when earth and sky were keeping a blithe holiday. But she was one of that meek sisterhood who, thinking humbly of themselves, believe they are honoured by being spent in the service of less conscientious souls, whose careless thanks seem quite reward enough.

To and fro she went, silent and diligent, giving the grace of willingness to every humble or distasteful task the day had brought her; but some malignant sprite seemed to have taken possession of her kingdom, for rebellion broke out everywhere. The kettles would boil over most obstreperously,—the mutton refused to cook with the meek alacrity to be expected from the nature of a sheep,—the stove, with unnecessary warmth of temper, would glow like a fiery furnace,—the irons would scorch,—the linens would dry,—and spirits would fail, though patience never.

Nan tugged on, growing hotter and wearier, more hurried and more hopeless, till at last the crisis came; for in one fell moment she tore her gown, burnt her hand, and smutched the collar she was preparing to finish in the most unexceptionable style. Then, if she had been a nervous woman, she would have scolded; being a gentle girl, she only "lifted up her voice and wept."

"Behold, she watereth her linen with salt tears, and bewaileth herself because of much tribulation. But, lo! Help cometh from afar: a strong man bringeth lettuce wherewith to stay her, pluckest berries to comfort her withal, and clasheth cymbals that she may dance for joy."

The voice came from the porch, and, with her hope fulfilled, Nan looked up to greet John Lord, the house-friend, who stood there with a basket on his arm; and as she saw his honest eyes, kind lips, and helpful hands, the girl thought this plain young man the comeliest, most welcome sight she had beheld that day.

"How good of you, to come through all this heat, and not to laugh at my despair!" she said, looking up like a grateful child, as she led him in.

"I only obeyed orders, Nan; for a certain dear old lady had a motherly presentiment that you had got into a domestic whirlpool, and sent me as a sort of life-preserver. So I took the basket of consolation, and came to fold my feet upon the carpet of contentment in the tent of friendship."

As he spoke, John gave his own gift in his mother's name, and bestowed himself in the wide window-seat, where morning-glories nodded at him, and the old butternut sent pleasant shadows dancing to and fro.

His advent, like that of Orpheus in Hades, seemed to soothe all unpropitious powers with a sudden spell. The fire began to slacken, the kettles began to lull, the meat began to cook, the irons began to cool, the clothes began to behave, the spirits began to rise, and the collar was finished off with most triumphant success. John watched the change, and, though a lord of creation, abased himself to take compassion on the weaker vessel, and was seized with a great desire to lighten the homely tasks that tried her strength of body and soul. He took a comprehensive glance about the room; then, extracting a dish from the closet, proceeded to imbrue his hands in the strawberries' blood.

"Oh, John, you needn't do that; I shall have time when I've turned the meat, made the pudding and done these things. See, I'm getting on finely now:—you're a judge of such matters; isn't that nice?"

As she spoke, Nan offered the polished absurdity for inspection with innocent pride.

"Oh that I were a collar, to sit upon that hand!" sighed John,—adding, argumentatively,

"As to the berry question, I might answer it with a gem from Dr. Watts, relative to 'Satan' and idle hands,' but will merely say, that, as a matter of public safety, you'd better leave me alone; for such is the destructiveness of my nature, that I shall certainly eat something hurtful, break something valuable, or sit upon something crushable, unless you let me concentrate my energies by knocking on these young fellows' hats, and preparing them for their doom."

Looking at the matter in a charitable light, Nan consented, and went cheerfully on with her work, wondering how she could have thought ironing an infliction, and been so ungrateful for the blessings of her lot.

"Where's Sally?" asked John, looking vainly for the functionary who usually pervaded that region like a domestic police-woman, a terror to cats, dogs, and men.

"She has gone to her cousin's funeral, and won't be back till Monday. There seems to be a great fatality among her relations; for one dies, or comes to grief in some way, about once a month. But I don't blame poor Sally for wanting to get away from this place now and then. I think I could find it in my heart to murder an imaginary friend or two, if I had to stay here long."

And Nan laughed so blithely, it was a pleasure to hear her.

"Where's Di?" asked John, seized with a most unmasculine curiosity all at once.

"She is in Germany with 'Wilhelm Meister'; but, though 'lost to sight, to memory dear'; for I was just thinking, as I did her things, how clever she is to like all kinds of books that I don't understand at all, and to write things that make me cry with pride and delight. Yes, she's a talented dear, though she hardly knows a needle from a crowbar, and will make herself one great blot some of these days, when the 'divine afflatus' descends upon her, I'm afraid."

And Nan rubbed away with sisterly zeal at Di's forlorn hose and inky pocket-handkerchiefs.

"Where is Laura?" proceeded the inquisitor.

"Well, I might say that she was in Italy; for she is copying some fine thing of Raphael's or Michel Angelo's, or some great creature's or other; and she looks so picturesque in her pretty gown, sitting before her easel, that it's really a sight to behold, and I've peeped two or three times to see how she gets on."

And Nan bestirred herself to prepare the dish Wherewith her picturesque sister desired to prolong her artistic existence.

"Where is your father?" John asked again, checking off each answer with a nod and a little frown.

"He is down in the garden, deep in some plan about melons, the beginning of which seems to consist in stamping the first proposition in Euclid all over the bed, and then poking a few seeds into the middle of each. Why, bless the dear man! I forgot it was time for the cider. Wouldn't you like to take it to him, John? He'd love to consult you; and the lane is so cool, it does one's heart good to look at it."

John glanced from the steamy kitchen to the shadowy path, and answered with a sudden assumption of immense industry,—

"I couldn't possibly go, Nan,—I've so much on my hands. You'll have to do it yourself. 'Mr. Robert of Lincoln' has something for your private ear; and the lane is so cool, it will do one's heart good to see you in it. Give my regards to your father, and, in the words of 'Little Mabel's' mother, with slight variation,—

'Tell the dear old body
This day I cannot run,
For the pots are boiling over
And the mutton isn't done.'"

"I will; but please, John, go in to the girls and be comfortable; for I don't like to leave you here," said Nan.

"You insinuate that I should pick at the pudding or invade the cream, do you? Ungrateful girl, leave me!" And, with melodramatic sternness, John extinguished her in his broad-brimmed hat, and offered the glass like a poisoned goblet.

Nan took it, and went smiling away. But the lane might have been the Desert of Sahara, for all she knew of it; and she would have passed her father as unconcernedly as if he had been an apple-tree, had he not called out,—

"Stand and deliver, little woman!"

She obeyed the venerable highwayman, and followed him to and fro, listening to his plans and directions with a mute attention that quite won his heart.

"That hop-pole is really an ornament now, Nan; this sage-bed needs weeding,—that's good work for you girls; and, now I think of it, you'd better water the lettuce in the cool of the evening, after I'm gone."

To all of which remarks Nan gave her assent; the hop-pole took the likeness of a tall figure she had seen in the porch, the sage-bed, curiously enough, suggested a strawberry ditto, the lettuce vividly reminded her of certain vegetable productions a basket had brought, and the bobolink only sung in his cheeriest voice, "Go home, go home! he is there!"

She found John—he having made a free-mason of himself, by assuming her little apron—meditating over the partially spread table, lost in amaze at its desolate appearance; one half its proper paraphernalia having been forgotten, and the other half put on awry. Nan laughed till the tears ran over her cheeks, and John was gratified at the efficacy of his treatment; for her face had brought a whole harvest of sunshine from the garden, and all her cares seemed to have been lost in the windings of the lane.

"Nan, are you in hysterics?" cried Di, appearing, book in hand. "John, you absurd man, what are you doing?"

"I'm helpin' the maid of all work, please marm." And John dropped a curtsy with his limited apron.

Di looked ruffled, for the merry words were a covert reproach; and with her usual energy of manner and freedom of speech she tossed "Wilhelm" out of the window, exclaiming, irefully,—

"That's always the way; I'm never where I ought to be, and never think of anything till it's too late; but it's all Goethe's fault. What does he write books full of smart 'Phillinas' and interesting 'Meisters' for? How can I be expected to remember that Sally's away, and people must eat, when I'm hearing the 'Harper' and little 'Mignon?' John, how dare you come here and do my work, instead of shaking me and telling me to do it myself? Take that toasted child away, and fan her like a Chinese mandarin, while I dish up this dreadful dinner."

John and Nan fled like chaff before the wind, while Di, full of remorseful zeal, charged at the kettles, and wrenched off the potatoes' jackets, as if she were revengefully pulling her own hair. Laura had a vague intention of going to assist; but, getting lost among the lights and shadows of Minerva's helmet, forgot to appear till dinner had been evoked from chaos and peace was restored.

At three o'clock, Di performed the coronation ceremony with her father's best hat; Laura retied his old-fashioned neckcloth, and arranged his white locks with an eye to saintly effect; Nan appeared with a beautifully written sermon, and suspicious ink-stains on the fingers that slipped it into his pocket; John attached himself to the bag; and the patriarch was escorted to the door of his tent with the triumphal procession which usually attended his out-goings and in-comings. Having kissed the female portion of his tribe, he ascended the venerable chariot, which received him with audible lamentation, as its rheumatic joints swayed to and fro.

"Good-bye, my dears! I shall be back early on Monday morning; so take care of yourselves, and be sure you all go and hear Mr. Emerboy preach to-morrow. My regards to your mother. John. Come, Solon!"

But Solon merely cocked one ear, and remained a fixed fact; for long experience had induced the philosophic beast to take for his motto the Yankee maxim, "Be sure you're right, then go ahead! He knew things were not right; therefore he did not go ahead.

"Oh, by the way, girls, don't forget to pay Tommy Mullein for bringing up the cow: he expects it to-night. And Di, don't sit up till daylight, nor let Laura stay out in the dew. Now, I believe I'm off. Come, Solon!"

But Solon only cocked the other ear, gently agitated his mortified tail, as premonitory symptoms of departure, and never stirred a hoof, being well aware that it always took three "comes" to make a "go."

"Bless me! I've forgotten my spectacles. They are probably shut up in that volume of Herbert on my table. Very awkward to find myself without them ten miles away. Thank you, John. Don't neglect to water the lettuce, Nan, and don't overwork yourself, my little 'Martha.' Come—"

At this juncture Solon suddenly went off, like "Mrs. Gamp," in a sort of walking swoon, apparently deaf and blind to all mundane matters, except the refreshments awaiting him ten miles away; and the benign old pastor disappeared, humming "Hebron" to the creaking accompaniment of the bulgy chaise.

Laura retired to take her siesta; Nan made a small *carbonaro* of herself by sharpening her sister's crayons, and Di, as a sort of penance for past sins, tried her patience over a piece of knitting, in which she soon originated a somewhat remarkable pattern, by dropping every third stitch, and seaming ad libitum. If John had been a gentlemanly creature, with refined tastes, he would have elevated his feet and made a nuisance of himself by indulging in a "weed;" but being only an uncultivated youth, with a rustic regard for pure air and womankind in general, he kept his head uppermost, and talked like a man, instead of smoking like a chimney.

"It will probably be six months before I sit here again, tangling your threads and maltreating your needles, Nan. How glad you must feel to hear it!" he said, looking up from a thoughtful examination of the hard-working little citizens of the Industrial Community settled in Nan's work-basket.

"No, I'm very sorry; for I like to see you coming and going as you used to, years ago, and I miss you very much when you are gone, John," answered truthful Nan, whittling away in a sadly wasteful manner, as her thoughts flew back to the happy times when a little lad rode a little lass in a big wheelbarrow, and never spilt his load,—when two brown heads bobbed daily side by side to school, and the favourite play was "Babes in the Wood," with Di for a somewhat peckish robin to cover the small martyrs with any vegetable substance that lay at hand. Nan sighed, as she thought of these things, and John regarded the battered thimble on his finger-tip with increased benignity of aspect as he heard the sound.

"When are you going to make your fortune, John, and get out of that disagreeable hardware concern?" demanded Di, pausing after an exciting "round," and looking almost as much exhausted as if it had been a veritable pugilistic encounter.

"I intend to make it by plunging still deeper into 'that disagreeable hardware concern;' for, next year, if the world keeps rolling, and John Lord is alive, he will become a partner, and then—and then—"

The colour sprang up into the young man's cheek, his eyes looked out with a sudden shine, and his hand seemed involuntarily to close, as if he saw and seized some invisible delight.

"What will happen then, John?" asked Nan, with a wondering glance.

"I'll tell you in a year, Nan, wait till then." and John's strong hand unclosed, as if the desired good were not to be his yet.

Di looked at him, with a knitting-needle stuck into her hair, saying, like a sarcastic unicorn,—

"I really thought you had a soul above pots and kettles, but I see you haven't; and I beg your pardon for the injustice I have done you."

Not a whit disturbed, John smiled, as if at some mighty pleasant fancy of his own, as he replied,—

"Thank you, Di; and as a further proof of the utter depravity of my nature, let me tell you that I have the greatest possible respect for those articles of ironmongery. Some of the happiest hours of my life have been spent in their society; some of my pleasantest associations are connected with them; some of my best lessons have come to me among them; and when my fortune is made, I intend to show my gratitude by taking three flat-irons rampant for my coat of arms."

Nan laughed merrily, as she looked at the burns on her hand; but Di elevated the most prominent feature of her brown countenance, and sighed despondingly,—

"Dear, dear, what a disappointing world this is! I no sooner build a nice castle in Spain, and settle a smart young knight therein, than down it comes about my ears; and the ungrateful youth, who might fight dragons, if he chose, insists on quenching his energies in a saucepan, and making a Saint Lawrence of himself by wasting his life on a series of gridirons. Ah, if I were only a man, I would do something better than that, and prove that heroes are not all dead yet. But, instead of that, I'm only a woman, and must sit rasping my temper with absurdities like this." And Di wrestled with her knitting as if it were Fate, and she were paying off the grudge she owed it.

John leaned toward her, saying, with a look that made his plain face handsome,—

"Di, my father began the world as I begin it, and left it the richer for the useful years he spent here,—as I hope I may leave it some half-century hence. His memory makes that dingy shop a pleasant place to me; for there he made an honest name, led an honest life and bequeathed to me his reverence for honest work. That is a sort of hardware, Di, that no rust can corrupt, and which will always prove a better fortune than any your knights can achieve with sword and shield. I think

I am not quite a clod, or quite without some aspirations above money-getting; for I sincerely desire that courage that makes daily life heroic by self-denial and cheerfulness of heart; I am eager to conquer my own rebellious nature, and earn the confidence of innocent and upright souls; I have a great ambition to become as good a man and leave as good a memory behind me as old John Lord."

Di winked violently, and seamed five times in perfect silence; but quiet Nan had the gift of knowing when to speak, and by a timely word saved her sister from a thunder-shower and her stocking from destruction.

"John, have you seen Philip since you wrote about your last meeting with him?"

The question was for John, but the soothing tone was for Di, who gratefully accepted it, and perked up again with speed.

"Yes; and I meant to have told you about it," answered John, plunging into the subject at once.

"I saw him a few days before I came home, and found him more disconsolate than ever,—'just ready to go to the Devil,' as he forcibly expressed himself. I consoled the poor lad as well as I could, telling him his wisest plan was to defer his proposed expedition, and go on as steadily as he had begun,—thereby proving the injustice of your father's prediction concerning his want of perseverance, and the sincerity of his affection. I told him the change in Laura's health and spirits was silently working in his favour, and that a few more months of persistent endeavour would conquer your father's prejudice against him, and make him a stronger man for the trial and the pain. I read him bits about Laura from your own and Di's letters, and he went away at last as patient as Jacob ready to serve another 'seven years' for his beloved Rachel."

"God bless you for it, John!" cried a fervent voice; and, looking up, they saw the cold, listless Laura transformed into a tender girl, all aglow with love and longing, as she dropped her mask, and showed a living countenance eloquent with the first passion and softened by the first grief of her life.

John rose involuntarily in the presence of an innocent nature whose sorrow needed no interpreter to him. The girl read sympathy in his brotherly regard, and found comfort in the friendly voice that asked, half playfully, half seriously,—

"Shall I tell him that he is not forgotten, even for an Apollo? that Laura the artist has not conquered Laura the woman? and predict that the good daughter will yet prove the happy wife?"

With a gesture full of energy, Laura tore her Minerva from top to bottom, while two great tears rolled down the cheeks grown wan with hope deferred.

"Tell him I believe all things, hope all things, and that I never can forget."

Nan went to her and held her fast, leaving the prints of two loving but grimy hands upon her shoulders; Di looked on approvingly, for, though stony-hearted regarding the cause, she fully appreciated the effect; and John, turning to the window, received the commendations of a robin swaying on an elm-bough with sunshine on its ruddy breast.

The clock struck five, and John declared that he must go; for, being an old-fashioned soul, he fancied that his mother had a better right to his last hour than any younger woman in the land,—always remembering that "she was a widow, and he her only son."

Nan ran away to wash her hands, and came back with the appearance of one who had washed her face also: and so she had; but there was a difference in the water.

"Play I'm your father, girls, and remember that it will be six months before 'that John' will trouble you again."

With which preface the young man kissed his former playfellows as heartily as the boy had been wont to do, when stern parents banished him to distant schools, and three little maids bemoaned his fate. But times were changed now; for Di grew alarmingly rigid during the ceremony; Laura received the salute like a graceful queen; and Nan returned it with heart and eyes and tender lips, making such an improvement on the child-ish fashion of the thing that John was moved to support his paternal character by softly echoing her father's words,—"Take care of yourself, my little 'Martha.'"

Then they all streamed after him along the garden-path, with the endless messages and warnings girls are so prone to give; and the young man, with a great soft-ness at his heart, went away, as many another John has gone, feeling better for the companionship of innocent maidenhood, and stronger to wrestle with temptation, to wait and hope and work.

"Let's throw a shoe after him for luck, as dear old 'Mrs. Gummage' did after 'David' and the 'willin' Barkis!' Quick, Nan! you always have old shoes on; toss one, and shout, 'Good luck!'" cried Di, with one of her eccentric inspirations.

Nan tore off her shoe, and threw it far along the dusty road, with a sudden longing to become that aus-picious article of apparel, that the omen might not fail.

Looking backward from the hill-top, John answered the meek shout cheerily, and took in the group with a lingering glance: Laura in the shadow of the elms, Di perched on the fence, and Nan leaning far over the gate with her hand above her eyes and the sunshine touching her brown hair with gold. He waved his hat and turned away; but the music seemed to die out of the blackbird's song, and in all the summer landscape his eyes saw nothing but the little figure at the gate.

"Bless and save us! here's a flock of people coming; my hair is in a toss, and Nan's without her shoe; run! fly, girls! or the Philistines will be upon us!" cried Di, tumbling off her perch in sudden alarm.

Three agitated young ladies, with flying draperies and countenances of mingled mirth and dismay, might have been seen precipitating themselves into a respectable mansion with unbecoming haste; but the squirrels were the only witnesses of this "vision of sudden flight," and, being used to ground-and-lofty tumbling, didn't mind it.

When the pedestrians passed, the door was decorously closed, and no one visible but a young man, who snatched something out of the road, and marched away again, whistling with more vigour of tone than accuracy of tune, "Only that, and nothing more."

HOW IT WAS FOUND

Summer ripened into autumn, and something fairer than

> "Sweet-peas and mignonette
> In Annie's garden grew."

Her nature was the counterpart of the hill-side grove, where as a child she had read her fairy tales, and now as a woman turned the first pages of a more wondrous legend still. Lifted above the many-gabled roof, yet not cut off from the echo of human speech, the little grove seemed a green sanctuary, fringed about with violets, and full of summer melody and bloom. Gentle creatures haunted it, and there was none to make afraid; wood-pigeons cooed and crickets chirped their shrill roundelays, anemones and lady-ferns looked up from the moss that kissed the wanderer's feet. Warm airs were all afloat, full of vernal odours for the grateful sense, silvery birches shimmered like spirits of the wood, larches gave their green tassels to the wind, and pines made airy music sweet and solemn, as they stood looking heavenward through veils of summer sunshine or shrouds of wintry snow.

Nan never felt alone now in this charmed wood; for when she came into its precincts, once so full of solitude, all things seemed to wear one shape, familiar eyes looked at her from the violets in the grass, familiar words sounded in the whisper of the leaves, grew conscious that an unseen influence filled the air with new delights, and touched earth and sky with a beauty never seen before. Slowly these Mayflowers budded in her maiden heart, rosily they bloomed and silently they waited till some lover of such lowly herbs should catch their fresh aroma, should brush away the fallen leaves, and lift them to the sun.

Though the eldest of the three, she had long been overtopped by the more aspiring maids. But though she meekly yielded the reins of government, whenever they chose to drive, they were soon restored to her again; for Di fell into literature, and Laura into love. Thus engrossed, these two forgot many duties which even bluestockings and innamoratas are expected to perform, and slowly all the homely humdrum cares that housewives know became Nan's daily life, and she accepted it without a thought of discontent. Noiseless and cheerful as the sunshine, she went to and fro, doing the tasks that mothers do, but without a mother's sweet reward, holding fast the numberless slight threads that bind a household tenderly together, and making each day a beautiful success.

Di, being tired of running, riding, climbing, and boating, decided at last to let her body rest and put her equally active mind through what classical collegians term "a course of sprouts." Having undertaken to read and know everything, she devoted herself to the task with great energy, going from Sue to Swedenborg with perfect impartiality, and having different authors as children have sundry distempers, being fractious while they lasted, but all the better for them when once over. Carlyle appeared like scarlet-fever, and raged violently for a time; for, being anything but a "passive bucket," Di became prophetic with Mahomet, belligerent with Cromwell, and made the French Revolution a veritable Reign of Terror to her family. Goethe and Schiller alternated like fever and ague; Mephistopheles became her hero, Joan of Arc her model, and she turned her black eyes red over Egmont and Wallenstein. A mild attack of Emerson followed, during which she was lost in a fog, and her sisters rejoiced inwardly when she emerged informing them that

> *"The Sphinx was drowsy,*
> *Her wings were furled."*

Poor Di was floundering slowly to her proper place; but she splashed up a good deal of foam by getting out of her depth, and rather exhausted herself by trying to drink the ocean dry.

Laura, after the "midsummer night's dream" that often comes to girls of seventeen, woke up to find that youth and love were no match for age and common sense. Philip had been flying about the world like a thistle-down for five-and-twenty years, generous-hearted, frank, and kind, but with never an idea of the serious side of life in his handsome head. Great, therefore, were the wrath and dismay of the enamoured thistle-down, when the father of his love mildly objected to seeing her begin the world in a balloon with a very tender but very inexperienced aeronaut for a guide.

"Laura is too young to 'play house' yet, and you are too unstable to assume the part of lord and master, Philip. Go and prove that you have prudence, patience, energy, and enterprise, and I will give you my girl,—but not before. I must seem cruel, that I may be truly kind; believe this, and let a little pain lead you to great happiness, or show you where you would have made a bitter blunder."

The lovers listened, owned the truth of the old man's words, bewailed their fate, and yielded,—Laura for love of her father, Philip for love of her. He went away to build a firm foundation for his castle in the air, and Laura retired into an invisible convent, where she cast off the world, and regarded her sympathizing sisters through a grate of superior knowledge and unsharable grief. Like a devout nun, she worshipped "St. Philip," and firmly believed in his miraculous powers. She fancied that her woes set her apart from common cares, and slowly fell into a dreamy state, professing no interest in any mundane matter, but the art that first attracted Philip. Crayons, bread-crusts, and grey paper became glorified in Laura's eyes; and her one pleasure was to sit pale and still before her easel, day after day, filling her portfolios with the faces he had once admired. Her sisters observed that every Bacchus, Piping Faun, or Dying Gladiator bore some likeness to a comely countenance that heathen god or hero never owned; and seeing this, they privately rejoiced that she had found such solace for her grief.

Mrs. Lord's keen eye had read a certain newly written page in her son's heart,—his first chapter of that romance, begun in paradise, whose interest never flags, whose beauty never fades, whose end can never come till Love lies dead. With womanly skill she divined the secret, with motherly discretion she counselled patience, and her son accepted her advice, feeling that, like many a healthful herb, its worth lay in its bitterness.

"Love like a man, John, not like a boy, and learn to know yourself before you take a woman's happiness into your keeping. You and Nan have known each other all your lives; yet, till this last visit, you never thought you loved her more than any other childish friend. It is too soon to say the words so often spoken hastily,—so hard to be recalled. Go back to your work, dear, for another year; think of Nan in the light of this new hope: compare her with comelier, gayer girls; and by absence prove the truth of your belief. Then, if distance only makes her dearer, if time only strengthens your affection, and no doubt of your own worthiness disturbs you, come back and offer her what any woman should be glad to take,—my boy's true heart."

John smiled at the motherly pride of her words, but answered with a wistful look.

"It seems very long to wait, mother. If I could just

ask her for a word of hope, I could be very patient then."

"Ah, my dear, better bear one year of impatience now than a lifetime of regret hereafter. Nan is happy; why disturb her by a word which will bring the tender cares and troubles that come soon enough to such conscientious creatures as herself? If she loves you, time will prove it; therefore, let the new affection spring and ripen as your early friendship has done, and it will be all the stronger for a summer's growth. Philip was rash, and has to bear his trial now, and Laura shares it with him. Be more generous, John; make your trial, bear your doubts alone, and give Nan the happiness without the pain. Promise me this, dear,—promise me to hope and wait."

The young man's eye kindled, and in his heart there rose a better chivalry, a truer valour, than any Di's knights had ever known.

"I'll try, mother," was all he said; but she was satisfied, for John seldom tried in vain.

"Oh, girls, how splendid you are! It does my heart good to see my handsome sisters in their best array," cried Nan, one mild October night, as she put the last touches to certain airy raiment fashioned by her own skilful hands, and then fell back to survey the grand effect.

"Di and Laura were preparing to assist at an event of the season," and Nan, with her own locks fallen on her shoulders, for want of sundry combs promoted to her sisters' heads and her dress in unwonted disorder, for lack of the many pins extracted in exciting crises of the toilet, hovered like an affectionate bee about two very full-blown flowers.

"Laura looks like a cool Undine, with the ivy-wreaths

in her shining hair; and Di has illuminated herself to such an extent with those scarlet leaves that I don't know what great creature she resembles most," said Nan, beaming with sisterly admiration.

"Like Juno, Zenobia, and Cleopatra simmered into one, with a touch of Xantippe by way of spice. But, to my eye, the finest woman of the three is the dishevelled young person embracing the bed-post: for she stays at home herself, and gives her time and taste to making homely people fine,—which is a waste of good material, and an imposition on the public."

As Di spoke, both the fashion-plates looked affectionately at the grey-gowned figure; but, being works of art, they were obliged to nip their feelings in the bud, and reserve their caresses till they returned to common life.

"Put on your bonnet, and we'll leave you at Mrs. Lord's on our way. It will do you good, Nan; and perhaps there may be news from John," added Di, as she bore down upon the door like a man-of-war under full sail.

"Or from Philip," sighed Laura, with a wistful look.

Whereupon Nan persuaded herself that her strong inclination to sit down was owing to want of exercise, and the heaviness of her eyelids a freak of imagination; so, speedily smoothing her ruffled plumage, she ran down to tell her father of the new arrangement.

"Go, my dear, by all means. I shall be writing; and you will be lonely if you stay. But I must see my girls; for I caught glimpses of certain surprising phantoms flitting by the door."

Nan led the way, and the two pyramids revolved before him with the rapidity of lay-figures, much to the good man's edification: for with his fatherly pleasure there was mingled much mild wonderment at the amplitude of array.

"Yes, I see my geese are really swans, though there is such a cloud between us that I feel a long way off, and hardly know them. But this little daughter is always available, always my 'cricket on the hearth.'"

As he spoke, her father drew Nan closer, kissed her tranquil face, and smiled content.

"Well, if ever I see picters, I see 'em now, and I declare to goodness it's as interestin' as playactin', every bit. Miss Di with all them boughs in her head, looks like the Queen of Sheby, when she went a-visitin' What's-his-name; and if Miss Laura ain't as sweet as a lally-barster figger, I should like to know what is."

In her enthusiasm, Sally gambolled about the girls, flourishing her milk-pan like a modern Miriam about to sound her timbrel for excess of joy.

Laughing merrily, the two Mont Blancs bestowed themselves in the family ark, Nan hopped up beside Patrick, and Solon, roused from his lawful slumbers, morosely trundled them away. But, looking backward with a last "Good-night!" Nan saw her father still standing at the door with smiling countenance, and the moonlight falling like a benediction on his silver hair.

"Betsey shall go up the hill with you, my dear, and here's a basket of eggs for your father. Give him my love, and be sure you let me know the next time he is poorly," Mrs. Lord said, when her guest rose to depart, after an hour of pleasant chat.

But Nan never got the gift; for, to her great dismay, her hostess dropped the basket with a crash, and flew across the room to meet a tall shape pausing in the shadow of the door. There was no need to ask who the new-comer was; for, even in his mother's arms, John looked over her shoulder with an eager nod to Nan, who stood among the ruins with never a sign of weariness in her face, nor the memory of a care at her heart,—for they all went out when John came in.

"Now tell us how and why and when you came. Take off your coat, my dear! And here are the old slippers. Why didn't you let us know you were coming so soon? How have you been? and what makes you so late to-night? Betsey, you needn't put on your bonnet. And—oh, my dear boy, have you been to supper yet?"

Mrs. Lord was a quiet soul, and her flood of questions was purred softly in her son's ear; for, being a woman, she must talk, and, being a mother, must pet the one delight of her life, and make a little festival when the lord of the manor came home. A whole drove of fatted calves were metaphorically killed, and a banquet appeared with speed.

John was not one of those romantic heroes who can go through three volumes of hair-breadth escapes without the faintest hint of that blessed institution, dinner; therefore, like "Lady Letherbridge," he partook, copiously of everything, while the two women beamed over each mouthful with an interest that enhanced its flavour, and urged upon him cold meat and cheese, pickles and pie, as if dyspepsia and nightmare were among the lost arts.

Then he opened his budget of news and fed them.

"I was coming next month, according to custom; but Philip fell upon and so tempted me, that I was driven to sacrifice myself to the cause of friendship, and up we came to-night. He would not let me come here till we had seen your father, Nan; for the poor lad was pining for Laura, and hoped his good behaviour for the past year would satisfy his judge and secure his recall. We had a fine talk with your father; and, upon my life, Philip seemed to have received the gift of tongues, for he made a most eloquent plea, which I've stored away for future use, I assure you. The dear old gentleman was very kind, told Phil he was satisfied with the success of his probation, that he should see Laura when he liked, and, if all went well, should receive his reward in the spring. It must be a delightful sensation to know you have made a fellow-creature as happy as those words made Phil to-night."

John paused, and looked musingly at the matronly tea-pot, as if he saw a wondrous future in its shine.

Nan twinkled off the drops that rose at the thought of Laura's joy, and said, with grateful warmth,—

"You say nothing of your own share in the making of that happiness, John; but we know it, for Philip has told Laura in his letters all that you have been to him, and I am sure there was other eloquence beside his own before father granted all you say he has. Oh, John, I thank you very much for this!"

Mrs. Lord beamed a whole midsummer of delight upon her son, as she saw the pleasure these words gave him, though he answered simply,—

"I only tried to be a brother to him, Nan; for he has been most kind to me. Yes, I said my little say to-night, and gave my testimony in behalf of the prisoner at the bar; a most merciful judge pronounced his sentence, and he rushed straight to Mrs. Leigh's to tell Laura the blissful news. Just imagine the scene when he appears, and how Di will open her wicked eyes and enjoy the spectacle of the dishevelled lover, the bride-elect's tears, the stir, and the romance of the thing. She'll cry over it to-night, and caricature it to-morrow."

And John led the laugh at the picture he had conjured

up, to turn the thoughts of Di's dangerous sister from himself.

At ten Nan retired into the depths of her old bonnet with a far different face from the one she brought out of it, and John, resuming his hat, mounted guard.

"Don't stay late, remember, John!" And in Mrs. Lord's voice there was a warning tone that her son interpreted aright.

"I'll not forget, mother."

And he kept his word; for though Philip's happiness floated temptingly before him, and the little figure at his side had never seemed so dear, he ignored the bland winds, the tender night, and set a seal upon his lips, thinking manfully within himself. "I see many signs of promise in her happy face; but I will wait and hope a little longer for her sake."

"Where is father, Sally?" asked Nan, as that functionary appeared, blinking owlishly, but utterly repudiating the idea of sleep.

"He went down the garding, miss, when the gentlemen cleared, bein' a little flustered by the goin's on. Shall I fetch him in?" asked Sally, as irreverently as if her master were a bag of meal.

"No, we will go ourselves." And slowly the two paced down the leaf-strewn walk.

Fields of yellow grain were waving on the hill-side, and sere corn blades rustled in the wind, from the orchard came the scent of ripening fruit, and all the garden-plots lay ready to yield up their humble offerings to their master's hand. But in the silence of the night a greater Reaper had passed by, gathering in the harvest of a righteous life, and leaving only tender memories for the gleaners who had come so late.

The old man sat in the shadow of the tree his own

hands planted; its fruit boughs shone ruddily, and its leaves still whispered the low lullaby that hushed him to his rest.

"How fast he sleeps! Poor father! I should have come before and made it pleasant for him."

As she spoke, Nan lifted up the head bent down upon his breast, and kissed his pallid cheek.

"Oh, John, this is not sleep."

"Yes, dear, the happiest he will ever know."

For a moment the shadows flickered over three white faces and the silence deepened solemnly. Then John reverently bore the pale shape in, and Nan dropped down beside it, saying, with a rain of grateful tears,—

"He kissed me when I went, and said a last good-night!'"

For an hour steps went to and fro about her, many voices whispered near her, and skilful hands touched the beloved clay she held so fast; but one by one the busy feet passed out, one by one the voices died away, and human skill proved vain.

Then Mrs. Lord drew the orphan to the shelter of her arms, soothing her with the mute solace of that motherly embrace.

"Nan, Nan! here's Philip! come and see!" The happy call re-echoed through the house, and Nan sprang up as if her time for grief were past.

"I must tell them. Oh, my poor girls, how will they bear it?—they have known so little sorrow!"

But there was no need for her to speak; other lips had spared her the hard task. For, as she stirred to meet them, a sharp cry rent the air, steps rang upon the stairs, and two wild-eyed creatures came into the hush of that familiar room, for the first time meeting with no welcome from their father's voice.

With one impulse, Di and Laura fled to Nan, and the sisters clung together in a silent embrace, more eloquent than words. John took his mother by the hand, and led her from the room, closing the door upon the sacredness of grief.

"Yes, we are poorer than we thought; but when everything is settled, we shall get on very well. We can let a part of this great house, and live quietly together until spring; then Laura will be married, and Di can go on their travels with them, as Philip wishes her to do. We shall be cared for; so never fear for us, John."

Nan said this, as her friend parted from her a week later, after the saddest holiday he had ever known.

"And what becomes of you, Nan?" he asked, watching the patient eyes that smiled when others would have wept.

"I shall stay in the dear old house; for no other place would seem like home to me. I shall find some little child to love and care for, and be quite happy till the girls come back and want me."

John nodded wisely, as he listened, and went away prophesying within himself,—

"She shall find something more than a child to love; and, God willing, shall be very happy till the girls come home and—cannot have her."

Nan's plan was carried into effect. Slowly the divided waters closed again, and the three fell back into their old life. But the touch of sorrow drew them closer; and, though invisible, a beloved presence still moved among them, a familiar voice still spoke to them in the silence of their softened hearts. Thus the soil was made ready, and in the depth of winter the good seed was sown, was watered with many tears, and soon sprang up green with a promise of a harvest for their after years.

Di and Laura consoled themselves with their favourite employments, unconscious that Nan was growing paler, thinner, and more silent, as the weeks went by, till one day she dropped quietly before them, and it suddenly became manifest that she was utterly worn out with many cares and the secret suffering of a tender heart bereft of the paternal love which had been its strength and stay.

"I'm only tired, dear girls. Don't be troubled, for I shall be up to-morrow," she said cheerily, as she looked into the anxious faces bending over her.

But the weariness was of many months' growth, and it was weeks before that "to-morrow" came.

Laura installed herself as nurse, and her devotion was repaid four-fold; for, sitting at her sister's bedside, she learned a finer art than that she had left. Her eye grew clear to see the beauty of a self-denying life, and in the depths of Nan's meek nature she found the strong, sweet virtues that made her what she was.

Then remembering that these womanly attributes were a bride's best dowry, Laura gave herself to their attainment, that she might become to another household the blessing Nan had been to her own; and turning from the worship of the goddess Beauty, she gave her hand to that humbler and more human teacher, Duty,—learning her lessons with a willing heart, for Philip's sake.

Di corked her inkstand, locked her bookcase, and went at housework as if it were a five-barred gate; of course she missed the leap, but scrambled bravely through, and appeared much sobered by the exercise. Sally had departed to sit under a vine and fig-tree of her own, so Di had undisputed sway; but if dish-pans and dusters had tongues, direful would have been the history of that crusade against frost and fire, indolence and inexperience. But they were dumb, and Di scorned to complain, though her struggles were pathetic to behold, and her sisters went through a series of messes equal to a course of "Prince Benreddin's" peppery tarts. Reality turned Romance out of doors; for, unlike her favourite heroines in satin and tears, or helmet and shield, Di met her fate in a big checked apron and dust-cap, wonderful to see; yet she wielded her broom as stoutly as "Moll Pitcher" shouldered her gun, and marched to her daily martyrdom in the kitchen with as heroic a heart as the "Maid of Orleans" took to her stake.

Mind won the victory over matter in the end, and Di was better all her days for the tribulations and the triumphs of that time; for she drowned her idle fancies in her wash-tub, made burnt-offerings of selfishness and pride, and learned the worth of self-denial, as she sang with happy voice among the pots and kettles of her conquered realm.

Nan thought of John, and in the stillness of her sleepless nights prayed Heaven to keep him safe, and make her worthy to receive and strong enough to bear the blessedness or pain of love.

Snow fell without, and keen winds howled among the leafless elms, but "herbs of grace" were blooming beautifully in the sunshine of sincere endeavour, and this dreariest season proved the most fruitful of the year; for love taught Laura, labour chastened Di, and patience fitted Nan for the blessing of her life.

Nature, that stillest, yet most diligent of housewives, began at last that "spring cleaning" which she makes so pleasant that none find the heart to grumble as they do when other matrons set their premises a-dust. Her hand-maids, wind and rain and sun, swept, washed, and garnished busily, green carpets were unrolled, apple-boughs were hung with draperies of bloom, and dandelions, pet nurslings of the year, came out to play upon the sward.

From the South returned that opera troupe whose manager is never in despair, whose tenor never sulks, whose prima donna never fails, and in the orchard bona fide matinees were held, to which buttercups and clovers crowded in their prettiest spring hats, and verdant young blades twinkled their dewy lorgnettes, as they bowed and made way for the floral belles.

May was bidding June good-morrow, and the roses were just dreaming that it was almost time to wake, when John came again into the quiet room which now seemed the Eden that contained his Eve. Of course there was a jubilee; but something seemed to have befallen the whole group, for never had they appeared in such odd frames of mind. John was restless, and wore an excited look, most unlike his usual serenity of aspect.

Nan the cheerful had fallen into a well of silence and was not to be extracted by any Hydraulic power, though she smiled like the June sky over her head. Di's peculiarities were out in full force, and she looked as if she would go off like a torpedo at a touch; but through all her moods there was a half-triumphant, half-remorseful expression in the glance she fixed on John. And Laura, once so silent, now sang like a blackbird, as she flitted to and fro; but her fitful song was always, "Philip, my king."

John felt that there had come a change upon the three, and silently divined whose unconscious influence had wrought the miracle. The embargo was off his tongue, and he was in a fever to ask that question which brings a flutter to the stoutest heart; but though the "man" had come, the "hour" had not. So, by way of steadying his nerves, he paced the room, pausing often to take notes of his companions, and each pause seemed to increase his wonder and content.

He looked at Nan. She was in her usual place, the rigid little chair she loved, because it once was large enough to hold a curly-headed playmate and herself. The old work-basket was at her side, and the battered thimble busily at work; but her lips wore a smile they had never worn before, the colour of the unblown roses touched her cheek, and her downcast eyes were full of light.

He looked at Di. The inevitable book was on her knee, but its leaves were uncut; the strong-minded knob of hair still asserted its supremacy aloft upon her head, and the triangular jacket still adorned her shoulders in defiance of all fashions, past, present, or to come; but the expression of her brown countenance had grown softer, her tongue had found a curb, and in her hand lay a card with "Potts, Kettel & Co." inscribed thereon, which she regarded with never a scornful word for the "Co."

He looked at Laura. She was before her easel as of old; but the pale nun had given place to a blooming girl, who sang at her work, which was no prim Pallas, but a Clytie turning her human face to meet the sun.

"John, what are you thinking of?"

He stirred as if Di's voice had disturbed his fancy at some pleasant pastime, but answered with his usual sincerity,—

"I was thinking of a certain dear old fairy tale called 'Cinderella.'"

"Oh!" said Di; and her "Oh" was a most impressive

monosyllable. "I see the meaning of your smile now; and though the application of the story is not very complimentary to all parties concerned, it is very just and very true."

She paused a moment, then went on with softened voice and earnest mien:—

"You think I am a blind and selfish creature. So I am, but not so blind and selfish as I have been; for many tears have cleared my eyes, and much sincere regret has made me humbler than I was. I have found a better book than any father's library can give me, and I have read it with a love and admiration that grew stronger as I turned the leaves. Henceforth I take it for my guide and gospel, and, looking back upon the selfish and neglectful past, can only say, Heaven bless your dear heart, Nan!"

Laura echoed Di's last words; for, with eyes as full of tenderness, she looked down upon the sister she had lately learned to know, saying, warmly,—

"Yes, 'Heaven bless your dear heart, Nan!' I never can forget all you have been to me; and when I am far away with Philip, there will always be one countenance more beautiful to me than any pictured face I may discover, there will be one place more dear to me than Rome. The face will be yours, Nan, always so patient, always so serene; and the dearer place will be this home of ours, which you have made so pleasant to me all these years by kindnesses as numberless and noiseless as the drops of dew."

"Dear girls, what have I ever done, that you should love me so?" cried Nan, with happy wonderment, as the tall heads, black and golden, bent to meet the lowly brown one, and her sisters' mute lips answered her.

Then Laura looked up, saying, playfully,—

"Here are the good and wicked sisters;—where shall we find the Prince?"

"There!" cried Di, pointing to John; and then her secret went off like a rocket; for, with her old impetuosity, she said,—

"I have found you out, John, and am ashamed to look you in the face, remembering the past. Girls, you know when father died, John sent us money, which he said Mr. Owen had long owed us and had paid at last? It was a kind lie, John, and a generous thing to do; for we needed it, but never would have taken it as a gift. I know you meant that we should never find this out; but yesterday I met Mr. Owen returning from the West, and when I thanked him for a piece of justice we had not expected of him, he gruffly told me he had never paid the debt, never meant to pay it, for it was outlawed, and we could not claim a farthing. John, I have laughed at you, thought you stupid, treated you unkindly; but I know you now, and never shall forget the lesson you have taught me. I am proud as Lucifer, but I ask you to forgive me, and I seal my real repentance so—and so."

With tragic countenance, Di rushed across the room, threw both arms about the astonished young man's neck and dropped an energetic kiss upon his cheek. There was a momentary silence; for Di finally illustrated her strong-minded theories by crying like the weakest of her sex. Laura, with "the ruling passion strong in death," still tried to draw, but broke her pet crayon, and endowed her Clytie with a supplementary orb, owing to the dimness of her own. And Nan sat with drooping eyes, that shone upon her work, thinking with tender pride,—"They know him now, and love him for his generous heart."

Di spoke first, rallying to her colours, though a little daunted by her loss of self-control.

"Don't laugh, John,—I couldn't help it; and don't think I'm not sincere, for I am,—I am; and I will prove it by growing good enough to be your friend. That debt must all be paid, and I shall do it; for I'll turn my books and pen to some account, and write stories full of clear old souls like you and Nan; and someone, I know, will like and buy them, though they are not 'works of Shakespeare.' I've thought of this before, have felt I had the power in me; now I have the motive, and now I'll do it."

If Di had proposed to translate the Koran, or build a new Saint Paul's, there would have been many chances of success; for, once moved, her will, like a battering-ram, would knock down the obstacles her wits could not surmount. John believed in her most heartily, and showed it, as he answered, looking into her resolute face,—

"I know you will, and yet make us very proud of our 'Chaos,' Di. Let the money lie, and when you have a fortune, I'll claim it with enormous interest; but, believe me, I feel already doubly repaid by the esteem so generously confessed, so cordially bestowed, and can only say, as we used to years ago,—Now let's forgive and so forget."

But proud Di would not let him add to her obligation, even by returning her impetuous salute; she slipped away, and, shaking off the last drops, answered with a curious mixture of old freedom and new respect,—

"No more sentiment, please, John. We know each other now; and when I find a friend, I never let him go. We have smoked the pipe of peace; so let us go back to our wigwams and bury the feud. Where were we when I lost my head? and what were we talking about?"

"Cinderella and the Prince."

As she spoke, John's eye kindled, and, turning, he looked down at Nan, who sat diligently ornamenting with microscopic stitches a great patch going on, the wrong side out.

"Yes,—so we were; and now taking pussy for the godmother, the characters of the story are well personated,—all but the slipper," said Di, laughing, as she thought of the many times they had played it together years ago.

A sudden movement stirred John's frame, a sudden purpose shone in his countenance, and a sudden change befell his voice, as he said, producing from some hiding-place a little worn-out shoe,—

"I can supply the slipper;—who will try it first?"

Di's black eyes opened wide, as they fell on the familiar object; then her romance-loving nature saw the whole plot of that drama which needs but two to act it. A great delight flushed up into her face, as she promptly took her cue, saying—

"No need for us to try it, Laura; for it wouldn't fit us, if our feet were as small as Chinese dolls; our parts are played out; therefore 'Exeunt wicked sisters to the music of the wedding-bells.'"

And pouncing upon the dismayed artist, she swept her out and closed the door with a triumphant bang.

John went to Nan, and, dropping on his knee as reverently as the herald of the fairy tale, he asked, still smiling, but with lips grown tremulous,—

"Will Cinderella try the little shoe, and—if it fits—go with the Prince?"

But Nan only covered up her face, weeping happy tears, while all the weary work strayed down upon the floor, as if it knew her holiday had come.

John drew the hidden face still closer, and while she listened to his eager words, Nan heard the beating of the strong man's heart, and knew it spoke the truth.

"Nan, I promised mother to be silent till I was sure I loved you wholly,—sure that the knowledge would give no pain when I should tell it, as I am trying to tell it now. This little shoe has been my comforter through this long year, and I have kept it as other lovers keep their fairer favours. It has been a talisman more eloquent to me than flower or ring; for, when I saw how worn it was, I always thought of the willing feet that came and went for others' comfort all day long; when I saw the little bow you tied, I always thought of the hands so diligent in serving anyone who knew a want or felt a pain; and when I recalled the gentle creature who had worn it last, I always saw her patient, tender, and devout,—and tried to grow more worthy of her, that I might one day dare to ask if she would walk beside me all my life and be my 'angel in the house.' Will you, dear? Believe me, you shall never know a weariness or grief I have the power to shield you from."

Then Nan, as simple in her love as in her life, laid her arms about his neck, her happy face against his own, and answered softly,—

"Oh, John, I never can be sad or tired anymore!"

Tobermory

It was a chill, rain-washed afternoon of a late August day, that indefinite season when partridges are still in security or cold storage, and there is nothing to hunt—unless one is bounded on the north by the Bristol Channel, in which case one may lawfully gallop after fat red stags. Lady Blemley's house-party was not bounded on the north by the Bristol Channel, hence there was a full gathering of her guests round the tea-table on this particular afternoon. And, in spite of the blankness of the season and the triteness of the occasion, there was no trace in the company of that fatigued restlessness which means a dread of the pianola and a subdued hankering for auction bridge. The undisguised open-mouthed attention of the entire party was fixed on the homely negative personality of Mr. Cornelius Appin. Of all her guests, he was the one who had come to Lady Blemley with the vaguest reputation. Someone had said he was "clever," and he had got his invitation in the moderate expectation, on the part of his hostess, that some portion at least of his cleverness would be contributed to the general entertainment. Until tea-time that day she had been unable to discover in what direction, if any, his cleverness lay. He was neither a wit nor a croquet champion, a hypnotic force nor a begetter of amateur theatricals. Neither did his exterior suggest the sort of man in whom women are willing to pardon a generous measure of mental deficiency. He had subsided into mere Mr. Appin, and the Cornelius seemed a piece of transparent baptismal bluff. And now he was claiming to have launched on the world a discovery beside which the invention of gunpowder, of the printing-press, and of steam locomotion were inconsiderable trifles. Science had made bewildering strides in many directions during recent decades, but this thing seemed to belong to the domain of miracle rather than to scientific achievement.

"And do you really ask us to believe," Sir Wilfrid was saying, "that you have discovered a means for instructing animals in the art of human speech, and that dear old Tobermory has proved your first successful pupil?"

"It is a problem at which I have worked for the last seventeen years," said Mr. Appin, "but only during the last eight or nine months have I been rewarded with glimmerings of success. Of course I have experimented with thousands of animals, but latterly only with cats, those wonderful creatures which have assimilated themselves so marvellously with our civilization while retaining all their highly developed feral instincts. Here and there among cats one comes across an outstanding superior intellect, just as one does among the ruck of human beings, and when I made the acquaintance of Tobermory a week ago I saw at once that I was in contact with a 'Beyond-cat' of extraordinary intelligence. I had gone far along the road to success in recent experiments; with Tobermory, as you call him, I have reached the goal."

Mr. Appin concluded his remarkable statement in a voice which he strove to divest of a triumphant inflection. No one said "Rats," though Clovis's lips moved in a monosyllabic contortion which probably invoked those rodents of disbelief.

"And do you mean to say," asked Miss Resker, after a slight pause, "that you have taught Tobermory to say and understand easy sentences of one syllable?"

"My dear Miss Resker," said the wonderworker patiently, "one teaches little children and savages and backward adults in that piecemeal fashion; when one has once solved the problem of making a beginning with an animal of highly developed intelligence one has no need for those halting methods. Tobermory can speak our language with perfect correctness."

This time Clovis very distinctly said, "Beyond-rats!" Sir Wilfrid was more polite, but equally sceptical.

"Hadn't we better have the cat in and judge for ourselves?" suggested Lady Blemley.

Sir Wilfrid went in search of the animal, and the company settled themselves down to the languid expectation of witnessing some more or less adroit drawing-room ventriloquism.

In a minute Sir Wilfrid was back in the room, his face white beneath its tan and his eyes dilated with excitement.

"By Gad, it's true!"

His agitation was unmistakably genuine, and his hearers started forward in a thrill of awakened interest.

Collapsing into an armchair he continued breathlessly: "I found him dozing in the smoking-room, and called out to him to come for his tea. He blinked at me in his usual way, and I said, 'Come on, Toby; don't keep us waiting;' and, by Gad! he drawled out in a most horribly natural voice that he'd come when he dashed well pleased! I nearly jumped out of my skin!"

Appin had preached to absolutely incredulous hearers; Sir Wilfrid's statement carried instant conviction. A Babel-like chorus of startled exclamation arose, amid which the scientist sat mutely enjoying the first fruit of his stupendous discovery.

In the midst of the clamour Tobermory entered the room and made his way with velvet tread and studied unconcern across to the group seated round the tea-table.

A sudden hush of awkwardness and constraint fell on the company. Somehow there seemed an element of embarrassment in addressing on equal terms a domestic cat of acknowledged dental ability.

"Will you have some milk, Tobermory?" asked Lady Blemley in a rather strained voice.

"I don't mind if I do," was the response, couched in a tone of even indifference. A shiver of suppressed excitement went through the listeners, and Lady Blemley might be excused for pouring out the saucerful of milk rather unsteadily.

"I'm afraid I've spilt a good deal of it," she said apologetically.

"After all, it's not my Axminster," was Tobermory's rejoinder.

Another silence fell on the group, and then Miss Resker, in her best district-visitor manner, asked if the human language had been difficult to learn. Tobermory looked squarely at her for a moment and then fixed his gaze serenely on the middle distance. It was obvious that boring questions lay outside his scheme of life.

"What do you think of human intelligence?" asked Mavis Pellington lamely.

"Of whose intelligence in particular?" asked Tobermory coldly.

"Oh, well, mine for instance," said Mavis, with a feeble laugh.

"You put me in an embarrassing position," said

Tobermory, whose tone and attitude certainly did not suggest a shred of embarrassment. "When your inclusion in this house-party was suggested Sir Wilfrid protested that you were the most brainless woman of his acquaintance, and that there was a wide distinction between hospitality and the care of the feeble-minded. Lady Blemley replied that your lack of brain-power was the precise quality which had earned you your invitation, as you were the only person she could think of who might be idiotic enough to buy their old car. You know, the one they call 'The Envy of Sisyphus,' because it goes quite nicely up-hill if you push it."

Lady Blemley's protestations would have had greater effect if she had not casually suggested to Mavis only that morning that the car in question would be just the thing for her down at her Devonshire home.

Major Barfield plunged in heavily to effect a diversion.

"How about your carryings-on with the tortoiseshell puss up at the stables, eh?"

The moment he had said it every one realized the blunder.

"One does not usually discuss these matters in public," said Tobermory frigidly. "From a slight observation of your ways since you've been in this house I should imagine you'd find it inconvenient if I were to shift the conversation on to your own little affairs."

The panic which ensued was not confined to the Major.

"Would you like to go and see if cook has got your dinner ready?" suggested Lady Blemley hurriedly, affecting to ignore the fact that it wanted at least two hours to Tobermory's dinner-time.

"Thanks," said Tobermory, "not quite so soon after my tea. I don't want to die of indigestion."

"Cats have nine lives, you know," said Sir Wilfrid heartily.

"Possibly," answered Tobermory; "but only one liver."

"Adelaide!" said Mrs. Cornett, "do you mean to encourage that cat to go out and gossip about us in the servants' hall?"

The panic had indeed become general. A narrow ornamental balustrade ran in front of most of the bedroom windows at the Towers, and it was recalled with dismay that this had formed a favourite promenade for Tobermory at all hours, whence he could watch the pigeons—and heaven knew what else besides. If he intended to become reminiscent in his present outspoken strain the effect would be something more than disconcerting. Mrs. Cornett, who spent much time at her toilet table, and whose complexion was reputed to be of a nomadic though punctual disposition, looked as ill at ease as the Major. Miss Scrawen, who wrote fiercely sensuous poetry and led a blameless life, merely displayed irritation; if you are methodical and virtuous in private you don't necessarily want every one to know it. Bertie van Tahn, who was so depraved at seventeen that he had long ago given up trying to be any worse, turned a dull shade of gardenia white, but he did not commit the error of dashing out of the room like Odo Finsberry, a young gentleman who was understood to be reading for the Church and who was possibly disturbed at the thought of scandals he might hear concerning other people. Clovis had the presence of mind to maintain a composed exterior; privately he was calculating how long it would take to procure a box of fancy mice through the agency of the Exchange and Mart as a species of hush-money.

Even in a delicate situation like the present, Agnes Resker could not endure to remain too long in the background.

"Why did I ever come down here?" she asked dramatically.

Tobermory immediately accepted the opening.

"Judging by what you said to Mrs. Cornett on the croquet-lawn yesterday, you were out for food. You described the Blemleys as the dullest people to stay with that you knew, but said they were clever enough to employ a first-rate cook; otherwise they'd find it difficult to get anyone to come down a second time."

"There's not a word of truth in it! I appeal to Mrs. Cornett—" exclaimed the discomfited Agnes.

"Mrs. Cornett repeated your remark afterwards to Bertie van Tahn," continued Tobermory, "and said, 'That woman is a regular Hunger Marcher; she'd go anywhere for four square meals a day,' and Bertie van Tahn said—"

At this point the chronicle mercifully ceased. Tobermory had caught a glimpse of the big yellow Tom from the Rectory working his way through the shrubbery towards the stable wing. In a flash he had vanished through the open French window.

With the disappearance of his too brilliant pupil Cornelius Appin found himself beset by a hurricane of bitter upbraiding, anxious inquiry, and frightened entreaty. The responsibility for the situation lay with him, and he must prevent matters from becoming worse. Could Tobermory impart his dangerous gift to other cats? was the first question he had to answer. It was possible, he replied, that he might have initiated his intimate friend the stable puss into his new accomplishment, but it was unlikely that his teaching could have taken a wider range as yet.

"Then," said Mrs. Cornett, "Tobermory may be a valuable cat and a great pet; but I'm sure you'll agree, Adelaide, that both he and the stable cat must be done away with without delay."

"You don't suppose I've enjoyed the last quarter of an hour, do you?" said Lady Blemley bitterly. "My husband and I are very fond of Tobermory—at least, we were before this horrible accomplishment was infused into him; but now, of course, the only thing is to have him destroyed as soon as possible."

"We can put some strychnine in the scraps he always gets at dinner-time," said Sir Wilfrid, "and I will go and drown the stable cat myself. The coachman will be very sore at losing his pet, but I'll say a very catching form of mange has broken out in both cats and we're afraid of it spreading to the kennels."

"But my great discovery!" expostulated Mr. Appin; "after all my years of research and experiment—"

"You can go and experiment on the shorthorns at the farm, who are under proper control," said Mrs. Cornett, "or the elephants at the Zoological Gardens. They're said to be highly intelligent, and they have this recommendation, that they don't come creeping about our bedrooms and under chairs, and so forth."

An archangel ecstatically proclaiming the Millennium, and then finding that it clashed unpardonably with Henley and would have to be indefinitely postponed, could hardly have felt more crestfallen than Cornelius Appin at the reception of his wonderful achievement. Public opinion, however, was against him—in fact, had the general voice been consulted on the subject it is probable that a strong minority vote would have been in favour of including him in the strychnine diet.

Defective train arrangements and a nervous desire to see matters brought to a finish prevented an immediate dispersal of the party, but dinner that evening was not a social success. Sir Wilfrid had had rather a trying time with the stable cat and subsequently with the coach-man. Agnes Resker ostentatiously limited her repast to a morsel of dry toast, which she bit as though it were a personal enemy; while Mavis Pellington maintained a vindictive silence throughout the meal. Lady Blemley kept up a flow of what she hoped was conversation, but her attention was fixed on the doorway. A plateful of carefully dosed fish scraps was in readiness on the side-board, but sweets and savoury and dessert went their way, and no Tobermory appeared either in the dining-room or kitchen.

The sepulchral dinner was cheerful compared with the subsequent vigil in the smoking-room. Eating and drinking had at least supplied a distraction and cloak to the prevailing embarrassment. Bridge was out of the question in the general tension of nerves and tempers, and after Odo Finsberry had given a lugubrious render-ing of "Melisande in the Wood" to a frigid audience, music was tacitly avoided. At eleven the servants went to bed, announcing that the small window in the pantry had been left open as usual for Tobermory's private use. The guests read steadily through the current batch of magazines, and fell back gradually, on the "Badminton Library" and bound volumes of PUNCH. Lady Blem-ley made periodic visits to the pantry, returning each time with an expression of listless depression which forestalled questioning.

At two o'clock Clovis broke the dominating silence.

"He won't turn up to-night. He's probably in the local newspaper office at the present moment, dictating the first instalment of his reminiscences. Lady What's-her-name's book won't be in it. It will be the event of the day."

Having made this contribution to the general cheerfulness, Clovis went to bed. At long intervals the various members of the house-party followed his example.

The servants taking round the early tea made a uniform announcement in reply to a uniform question. Tobermory had not returned.

Breakfast was, if anything, a more unpleasant function than dinner had been, but before its conclusion the situation was relieved. Tobermory's corpse was brought in from the shrubbery, where a gardener had just discovered it. From the bites on his throat and the yellow fur which coated his claws it was evident that he had fallen in unequal combat with the big Tom from the Rectory.

By midday most of the guests had quitted the Towers, and after lunch Lady Blemley had sufficiently recovered her spirits to write an extremely nasty letter to the Rectory about the loss of her valuable pet.

Tobermory had been Appin's one successful pupil, and he was destined to have no successor. A few weeks later an elephant in the Dresden Zoological Garden, which had shown no previous signs of irritability, broke loose and killed an Englishman who had apparently been teasing it. The victim's name was variously reported in the papers as Oppin and Eppelin, but his front name was faithfully rendered Cornelius.

"If he was trying German irregular verbs on the poor beast," said Clovis, "he deserved all he got."

Kew Gardens

From the oval-shaped flower-bed there rose perhaps a hundred stalks spreading into heart-shaped or tongue-shaped leaves half way up and unfurling at the tip red or blue or yellow petals marked with spots of colour raised upon the surface; and from the red, blue or yellow gloom of the throat emerged a straight bar, rough with gold dust and slightly clubbed at the end. The petals were voluminous enough to be stirred by the summer breeze, and when they moved, the red, blue and yellow lights passed one over the other, staining an inch of the brown earth beneath with a spot of the most intricate colour. The light fell either upon the smooth, grey back of a pebble, or, the shell of a snail with its brown, circular veins, or falling into a raindrop, it expanded with such intensity of red, blue and yellow the thin walls of water that one expected them to burst and disappear. Instead, the drop was left in a second silver grey once more, and the light now settled upon the flesh of a leaf, revealing the branching thread of fibre beneath the surface, and again it moved on and spread its illumination in the vast green spaces beneath the dome of the heart-shaped and tongue-shaped leaves. Then the breeze stirred rather more briskly overhead and the colour was flashed into the air above, into the eyes of the men and women who walk in Kew Gardens in July.

The figures of these men and women straggled past the flower-bed with a curiously irregular movement not unlike that of the white and blue butterflies who crossed the turf in zig-zag flights from bed to bed. The man was about six inches in front of the woman, strolling carelessly, while she bore on with greater purpose, only turning her head now and then to see that the children were not too far behind. The man kept this distance in front of the woman purposely, though perhaps unconsciously, for he wished to go on with his thoughts.

"Fifteen years ago I came here with Lily," he thought. "We sat somewhere over there by a lake and I begged her to marry me all through the hot afternoon. How the dragonfly kept circling round us: how clearly I see the dragonfly and her shoe with the square silver buckle at the toe. All the time I spoke I saw her shoe and when it moved impatiently I knew without looking up what she was going to say: the whole of her seemed to be in her shoe. And my love, my desire, were in the dragonfly; for some reason I thought that if it settled there, on that leaf, the broad one with the red flower in the middle of it, if the dragonfly settled on the leaf she would say 'Yes' at once. But the dragonfly went round and round: it never settled anywhere—of course not, happily not, or I shouldn't be walking here with Eleanor and the children—Tell me, Eleanor. D'you ever think of the past?"

"Why do you ask, Simon?"

"Because I've been thinking of the past. I've been thinking of Lily, the woman I might have married . . . Well, why are you silent? Do you mind my thinking of the past?"

"Why should I mind, Simon? Doesn't one always think of the past, in a garden with men and women lying under the trees? Aren't they one's past, all that remains of it, those men and women, those ghosts lying under the trees, . . . one's happiness, one's reality?"

"For me, a square silver shoe buckle and a dragonfly—"

"For me, a kiss. Imagine six little girls sitting before their easels twenty years ago, down by the side of a lake, painting the water-lilies, the first red water-lilies I'd ever seen. And suddenly a kiss, there on the back of my neck. And my hand shook all the afternoon so that I couldn't paint. I took out my watch and marked the hour when I would allow myself to think of the kiss for five minutes only—it was so precious—the kiss of an old grey-haired woman with a wart on her nose, the mother of all my kisses all my life. Come, Caroline, come, Hubert."

They walked on past the flower-bed, now walking four abreast, and soon diminished in size among the trees and looked half transparent as the sunlight and shade swam over their backs in large trembling irregular patches.

In the oval flower bed the snail, whose shell had been stained red, blue, and yellow for the space of two minutes or so, now appeared to be moving very slightly in its shell, and next began to labour over the crumbs of loose earth which broke away and rolled down as it passed over them. It appeared to have a definite goal in front of it, differing in this respect from the singular high stepping angular green insect who attempted to cross in front of it, and waited for a second with its antennæ trembling as if in deliberation, and then stepped off as rapidly and strangely in the opposite direction. Brown cliffs with deep green lakes in the hollows, flat, blade-like trees that waved from root to tip, round boulders of grey stone, vast crumpled surfaces of a thin crackling texture—all these objects lay across the snail's progress between one stalk and another to his goal. Before he had decided whether to circumvent the arched tent of a dead leaf or to breast it there came past the bed the feet of other human beings.

This time they were both men. The younger of the two wore an expression of perhaps unnatural calm; he raised his eyes and fixed them very steadily in front of him while his companion spoke, and directly his companion had done speaking he looked on the ground again and sometimes opened his lips only after a long pause and sometimes did not open them at all. The elder man had a curiously uneven and shaky method of walking, jerking his hand forward and throwing up his head abruptly, rather in the manner of an impatient carriage horse tired of waiting outside a house; but in the man these gestures were irresolute and pointless. He talked almost incessantly; he smiled to himself and again began to talk, as if the smile had been an answer. He was talking about spirits—the spirits of the dead, who, according to him, were even now telling him all sorts of odd things about their experiences in Heaven.

"Heaven was known to the ancients as Thessaly, William, and now, with this war, the spirit matter is rolling between the hills like thunder." He paused, seemed to listen, smiled, jerked his head and continued:—

"You have a small electric battery and a piece of rubber to insulate the wire—isolate?—insulate?—well, we'll skip the details, no good going into details that wouldn't be understood—and in short the little machine stands in any convenient position by the head of the bed, we will say, on a neat mahogany stand. All arrangements being properly fixed by workmen under my direction, the widow applies her ear and summons the spirit by sign as agreed. Women! Widows! Women in black—"

Here he seemed to have caught sight of a woman's dress in the distance, which in the shade looked a purple black. He took off his hat, placed his hand upon his heart, and hurried towards her muttering and gesticulating feverishly. But William caught him by the sleeve and touched a flower with the tip of his walking-stick in order to divert the old man's attention. After looking at it for a moment in some confusion the old man bent his ear to it and seemed to answer a voice speaking from it, for he began talking about the forests of Uruguay which he had visited hundreds of years ago in company with the most beautiful young woman in Europe. He could be heard murmuring about forests of Uruguay blanketed with the wax petals of tropical roses, nightingales, sea beaches, mermaids, and women drowned at sea, as he suffered himself to be moved on by William, upon whose face the look of stoical patience grew slowly deeper and deeper.

Following his steps so closely as to be slightly puzzled by his gestures came two elderly women of the lower middle class, one stout and ponderous, the other rosy cheeked and nimble. Like most people of their station they were frankly fascinated by any signs of eccentricity betokening a disordered brain, especially in the well-to-do; but they were too far off to be certain whether the gestures were merely eccentric or genuinely mad. After they had scrutinised the old man's back in silence for a moment and given each other a queer, sly look, they went on energetically piecing together their very complicated dialogue:

"Nell, Bert, Lot, Cess, Phil, Pa, he says, I says, she says, I says, I says, I says—"

"My Bert, Sis, Bill, Grandad, the old man, sugar,

Sugar, flour, kippers, greens,
Sugar, sugar, sugar."

The ponderous woman looked through the pattern of falling words at the flowers standing cool, firm, and upright in the earth, with a curious expression. She saw them as a sleeper waking from a heavy sleep sees a brass candlestick reflecting the light in an unfamiliar way, and closes his eyes and opens them, and seeing the brass candlestick again, finally starts broad awake and stares at the candlestick with all his powers. So the heavy woman came to a standstill opposite the oval-shaped flower bed, and ceased even to pretend to listen to what the other woman was saying. She stood there letting the words fall over her, swaying the top part of her body slowly backwards and forwards, looking at the flowers. Then she suggested that they should find a seat and have their tea.

The snail had now considered every possible method of reaching his goal without going round the dead leaf or climbing over it. Let alone the effort needed for climbing a leaf, he was doubtful whether the thin texture which vibrated with such an alarming crackle when touched even by the tip of his horns would bear his weight; and this determined him finally to creep beneath it, for there was a point where the leaf curved high enough from the ground to admit him. He had just inserted his head in the opening and was taking stock of the high brown roof and was getting used to the cool brown light when two other people came past outside on the turf. This time they were both young, a young man and a young woman. They were both in the prime of youth, or even in that season which precedes the prime of youth, the season before the smooth pink folds of the flower have burst their gummy case, when the wings of the butterfly, though fully grown, are motionless in the sun.

"Lucky it isn't Friday," he observed.

"Why? D'you believe in luck?"

"They make you pay sixpence on Friday."

"What's sixpence anyway? Isn't it worth sixpence?"

"What's 'it'—what do you mean by 'it'?"

"O, anything—I mean—you know what I mean."

Long pauses came between each of these remarks; they were uttered in toneless and monotonous voices. The couple stood still on the edge of the flower bed, and together pressed the end of her parasol deep down into the soft earth. The action and the fact that his hand rested on the top of hers expressed their feelings in a strange way, as these short insignificant words also expressed something, words with short wings for their heavy body of meaning, inadequate to carry them far and thus alighting awkwardly upon the very common objects that surrounded them, and were to their inexperienced touch so massive; but who knows (so they thought as they pressed the parasol into the earth) what precipices aren't concealed in them, or what slopes of ice don't shine in the sun on the other side? Who knows? Who has ever seen this before? Even when she wondered what sort of tea they gave you at Kew, he felt that something loomed up behind her words, and stood vast and solid behind them; and the mist very slowly rose and uncovered—O, Heavens, what were those shapes?—little white tables, and waitresses who looked first at her and then at him; and there was a bill that he would pay with a real two shilling piece, and it was real, all real, he assured himself, fingering the coin in his pocket, real to everyone except to him and to her; even to him it began to seem real; and then—but it was too exciting to stand and think any longer, and he pulled the parasol out of the earth with a jerk and was impatient to find the place where one had tea with other people, like other people.

"Come along, Trissie; it's time we had our tea."

"Wherever *does* one have one's tea?" she asked with the oddest thrill of excitement in her voice, looking vaguely round and letting herself be drawn on down the grass path, trailing her parasol, turning her head this way and that way, forgetting her tea, wishing to go down there and then down there, remembering orchids and cranes among wild flowers, a Chinese pagoda and a crimson crested bird; but he bore her on.

Thus one couple after another with much the same irregular and aimless movement passed the flower-bed and were enveloped in layer after layer of green blue vapour, in which at first their bodies had substance and a dash of colour, but later both substance and colour dissolved in the green-blue atmosphere. How hot it was! So hot that even the thrush chose to hop, like a mechanical bird, in the shadow of the flowers, with long pauses between one movement and the next; instead of rambling vaguely the white butterflies danced one above another, making with their white shifting flakes the outline of a shattered marble column above the tallest flowers; the glass roofs of the palm house shone as if a whole market full of shiny green umbrellas had opened in the sun; and in the drone of the aeroplane the voice of the summer sky murmured its fierce soul. Yellow and black, pink and snow white, shapes of all these colours, men, women, and children were spotted for a second upon the horizon, and then, seeing the breadth of yellow that lay upon the grass, they wavered and sought shade beneath the trees, dissolving like drops of water in the yellow and green atmosphere, staining it faintly with red and blue. It seemed as if all gross and heavy bodies had sunk down in the heat motionless and lay huddled upon the ground, but their voices went wavering from them as if they were flames lolling from the thick waxen bodies of candles. Voices. Yes, voices. Wordless voices, breaking the silence suddenly with such depth of contentment, such passion of desire, or, in the voices of children, such freshness of surprise; breaking the silence? But there was no silence; all the time the motor omnibuses were turning their wheels and changing their gear; like a vast nest of Chinese boxes all of wrought steel turning ceaselessly one within another the city murmured; on the top of which the voices cried aloud and the petals of myriads of flowers flashed their colours into the air.

F. SCOTT FITZGERALD

Head and Shoulders

I

In 1915 Horace Tarbox was thirteen years old. In that year he took the examinations for entrance to Princeton University and received the Grade A—excellent—in Caesar, Cicero, Vergil, Xenophon, Homer, Algebra, Plane Geometry, Solid Geometry, and Chemistry.

Two years later while George M. Cohan was composing "Over There," Horace was leading the sophomore class by several lengths and digging out theses on "The Syllogism as an Obsolete Scholastic Form," and during the battle of Chateau-Thierry he was sitting at his desk deciding whether or not to wait until his seventeenth birthday before beginning his series of essays on "The Pragmatic Bias of the New Realists."

After a while some newsboy told him that the war was over, and he was glad, because it meant that Peat Brothers, publishers, would get out their new edition of "Spinoza's Improvement of the Understanding." Wars were all very well in their way, made young men self-reliant or something, but Horace felt that he could never forgive the President for allowing a brass band to play under his window the night of the false armistice, causing him to leave three important sentences out of his thesis on "German Idealism."

The next year he went up to Yale to take his degree as Master of Arts.

He was seventeen then, tall and slender, with near-sighted grey eyes and an air of keeping himself utterly detached from the mere words he let drop.

"I never feel as though I'm talking to him," expostulated Professor Dillinger to a sympathetic colleague. "He makes me feel as though I were talking to his representative. I always expect him to say: 'Well, I'll ask myself and find out.'"

And then, just as nonchalantly as though Horace Tarbox had been Mr. Beef the butcher or Mr. Hat the haberdasher, life reached in, seized him, handled him, stretched him, and unrolled him like a piece of Irish lace on a Saturday-afternoon bargain-counter.

To move in the literary fashion I should say that this was all because when way back in colonial days the hardy pioneers had come to a bald place in Connecticut and asked of each other, "Now, what shall we build here?" the hardiest one among 'em had answered: "Let's build a town where theatrical managers can try out musical comedies!" How afterward they founded Yale College there, to try the musical comedies on, is a story everyone knows. At any rate one December, "Home James" opened at the Shubert, and all the students encored Marcia Meadow, who sang a song about the Blundering Blimp in the first act and did a shaky, shivery, celebrated dance in the last.

Marcia was nineteen. She didn't have wings, but audiences agreed generally that she didn't need them. She was a blonde by natural pigment, and she wore no paint on the streets at high noon. Outside of that she was no better than most women.

It was Charlie Moon who promised her five thousand Pall Malls if she would pay a call on Horace Tarbox, prodigy extraordinary. Charlie was a senior in

Sheffield, and he and Horace were first cousins. They liked and pitied each other.

Horace had been particularly busy that night. The failure of the Frenchman Laurier to appreciate the significance of the new realists was preying on his mind. In fact, his only reaction to a low, clear-cut rap at his study was to make him speculate as to whether any rap would have actual existence without an ear there to hear it. He fancied he was verging more and more toward pragmatism. But at that moment, though he did not know it, he was verging with astounding rapidity toward something quite different.

The rap sounded—three seconds leaked by—the rap sounded.

"Come in," muttered Horace automatically.

He heard the door open and then close, but, bent over his book in the big armchair before the fire, he did not look up.

"Leave it on the bed in the other room," he said absently.

"Leave what on the bed in the other room?"

Marcia Meadow had to talk her songs, but her speaking voice was like byplay on a harp.

"The laundry."

"I can't."

Horace stirred impatiently in his chair.

"Why can't you?"

"Why, because I haven't got it."

"Hm!" he replied testily. "Suppose you go back and get it."

Across the fire from Horace was another easy chair. He was accustomed to change to it in the course of an evening by way of exercise and variety. One chair he called Berkeley, the other he called Hume. He suddenly heard a sound as of a rustling, diaphanous form sinking into Hume. He glanced up.

"Well," said Marcia with the sweet smile she used in Act Two ("Oh, so the Duke liked my dancing!") "Well, Omar Khayyam, here I am beside you singing in the wilderness."

Horace stared at her dazedly. The momentary suspicion came to him that she existed there only as a phantom of his imagination. Women didn't come into men's rooms and sink into men's Humes. Women brought laundry and took your seat in the street-car and married you later on when you were old enough to know fetters.

This woman had clearly materialised out of Hume. The very froth of her brown gauzy dress was an emanation from Hume's leather arm there! If he looked long enough he would see Hume right through her and then he would be alone again in the room. He passed his fist across his eyes. He really must take up those trapeze exercises again.

"For Pete's sake, don't look so critical!" objected the emanation pleasantly. "I feel as if you were going to wish me away with that patent dome of yours. And then there wouldn't be anything left of me except my shadow in your eyes."

Horace coughed. Coughing was one of his two gestures. When he talked you forgot he had a body at all. It was like hearing a phonograph record by a singer who had been dead a long time.

"What do you want?" he asked.

"I want them letters," whined Marcia melodramatically—"them letters of mine you bought from my grandsire in 1881."

Horace considered.

"I haven't got your letters," he said evenly. "I am only seventeen years old. My father was not born until March 3, 1879. You evidently have me confused with someone else."

"You're only seventeen?" repeated March suspiciously.

"Only seventeen."

"I knew a girl," said Marcia reminiscently, "who went on the ten-twenty-thirty when she was sixteen. She was so stuck on herself that she could never say 'sixteen' without putting the 'only' before it. We got to calling her 'Only Jessie.' And she's just where she was when she started—only worse. 'Only' is a bad habit, Omar—it sounds like an alibi."

"My name is not Omar."

"I know," agreed Marcia, nodding—"your name's Horace. I just call you Omar because you remind me of a smoked cigarette."

"And I haven't your letters. I doubt if I've ever met your grandfather. In fact, I think it very improbable that you yourself were alive in 1881."

Marcia stared at him in wonder.

"Me—1881? Why sure! I was second-line stuff when the Florodora Sextette was still in the convent. I was the original nurse to Mrs. Sol Smith's Juliette. Why, Omar, I was a canteen singer during the War of 1812."

Horace's mind made a sudden successful leap, and he grinned.

"Did Charlie Moon put you up to this?"

Marcia regarded him inscrutably.

"Who's Charlie Moon?"

"Small—wide nostrils—big ears."

She grew several inches and sniffed.

"I'm not in the habit of noticing my friends' nostrils."

"Then it was Charlie?"

Marcia bit her lip—and then yawned. "Oh, let's change the subject, Omar. I'll pull a snore in this chair in a minute."

"Yes," replied Horace gravely, "Hume has often been considered soporific—"

"Who's your friend—and will he die?"

Then of a sudden Horace Tarbox rose slenderly and began to pace the room with his hands in his pockets. This was his other gesture.

"I don't care for this," he said as if he were talking to himself—"at all. Not that I mind your being here—I don't. You're quite a pretty little thing, but I don't like Charlie Moon's sending you up here. Am I a laboratory experiment on which the janitors as well as the chemists can make experiments? Is my intellectual development humorous in any way? Do I look like the pictures of the little Boston boy in the comic magazines? Has that callow ass, Moon, with his eternal tales about his week in Paris, any right to—"

"No," interrupted Marcia emphatically. "And you're a sweet boy. Come here and kiss me."

Horace stopped quickly in front of her.

"Why do you want me to kiss you?" he asked intently, "Do you just go round kissing people?"

"Why, yes," admitted Marcia, unruffled. "'At's all life is. Just going round kissing people."

"Well," replied Horace emphatically, "I must say your ideas are horribly garbled! In the first place life isn't just that, and in the second place I won't kiss you. It might get to be a habit and I can't get rid of habits. This year I've got in the habit of lolling in bed until seven-thirty—"

Marcia nodded understandingly.

"Do you ever have any fun?" she asked.

"What do you mean by fun?"

"See here," said Marcia sternly, "I like you, Omar, but I wish you'd talk as if you had a line on what you were saying. You sound as if you were gargling a lot of words in your mouth and lost a bet every time you spilled a few. I asked you if you ever had any fun."

Horace shook his head.

"Later, perhaps," he answered. "You see I'm a plan. I'm an experiment. I don't say that I don't get tired of it sometimes—I do. Yet—oh, I can't explain! But what you and Charlie Moon call fun wouldn't be fun to me."

"Please explain."

Horace stared at her, started to speak and then, changing his mind, resumed his walk. After an unsuccessful attempt to determine whether or not he was looking at her Marcia smiled at him.

"Please explain."

Horace turned.

"If I do, will you promise to tell Charlie Moon that I wasn't in?"

"Uh-uh."

"Very well, then. Here's my history: I was a 'why' child. I wanted to see the wheels go round. My father was a young economics professor at Princeton. He brought me up on the system of answering every question I asked him to the best of his ability. My response to that gave him the idea of making an experiment in precocity. To aid in the massacre I had ear trouble—seven operations between the age of nine and twelve. Of course this kept me apart from other boys and made me ripe for forcing. Anyway, while my generation was labouring through Uncle Remus I was honestly enjoying Catullus in the original.

"I passed off my college examinations when I was

thirteen because I couldn't help it. My chief associates were professors, and I took a tremendous pride in knowing that I had a fine intelligence, for though I was unusually gifted I was not abnormal in other ways. When I was sixteen I got tired of being a freak; I decided that someone had made a bad mistake. Still as I'd gone that far I concluded to finish it up by taking my degree of Master of Arts. My chief interest in life is the study of modern philosophy. I am a realist of the School of Anton Laurier—with Bergsonian trimmings—and I'll be eighteen years old in two months. That's all."

"Whew!" exclaimed Marcia. "That's enough! You do a neat job with the parts of speech."

"Satisfied?"

"No, you haven't kissed me."

"It's not in my programme," demurred Horace. "Understand that I don't pretend to be above physical things. They have their place, but—"

"Oh, don't be so darned reasonable!"

"I can't help it."

"I hate these slot-machine people."

"I assure you I—" began Horace.

"Oh shut up!"

"My own rationality—"

"I didn't say anything about your nationality. You're Amuricun, ar'n't you?"

"Yes."

"Well, that's O.K. with me. I got a notion I want to see you do something that isn't in your highbrow pro- gramme. I want to see if a what-ch-call-em with Brazil- ian trimmings—that thing you said you were—can be a little human."

Horace shook his head again.

"I won't kiss you."

"My life is blighted," muttered Marcia tragically. "I'm a beaten woman. I'll go through life without ever having a kiss with Brazilian trimmings." She sighed. "Anyways, Omar, will you come and see my show?"

"What show?"

"I'm a wicked actress from 'Home James'!"

"Light opera?"

"Yes—at a stretch. One of the characters is a Brazilian rice-planter. That might interest you."

"I saw 'The Bohemian Girl' once," reflected Horace aloud. "I enjoyed it—to some extent—"

"Then you'll come?"

"Well, I'm—I'm—"

"Oh, I know—you've got to run down to Brazil for the week-end."

"Not at all. I'd be delighted to come—"

Marcia clapped her hands.

"Goodyforyou! I'll mail you a ticket—Thursday night?"

"Why, I—"

"Good! Thursday night it is."

She stood up and walking close to him laid both hands on his shoulders.

"I like you, Omar. I'm sorry I tried to kid you. I thought you'd be sort of frozen, but you're a nice boy."

He eyed her sardonically.

"I'm several thousand generations older than you are."

"You carry your age well."

They shook hands gravely.

"My name's Marcia Meadow," she said emphatically. "'Member it—Marcia Meadow. And I won't tell Charlie Moon you were in."

An instant later as she was skimming down the last flight of stairs three at a time she heard a voice call over the upper banister: "Oh, say—"

She stopped and looked up—made out a vague form leaning over.

"Oh, say!" called the prodigy again. "Can you hear me?"

"Here's your connection Omar."

"I hope I haven't given you the impression that I consider kissing intrinsically irrational."

"Impression? Why, you didn't even give me the kiss! Never fret—so long."

Two doors near her opened curiously at the sound of a feminine voice. A tentative cough sounded from above. Gathering her skirts, Marcia dived wildly down the last flight, and was swallowed up in the murky Connecticut air outside.

Up-stairs Horace paced the floor of his study. From time to time he glanced toward Berkeley waiting there in suave dark-red reputability, an open book lying suggestively on his cushions. And then he found that his circuit of the floor was bringing him each time nearer to Hume. There was something about Hume that was strangely and inexpressibly different. The diaphanous form still seemed hovering near, and had Horace sat there he would have felt as if he were sitting on a lady's lap. And though Horace couldn't have named the quality of difference, there was such a quality—quite intangible to the speculative mind, but real, nevertheless. Hume was radiating something that in all the two hundred years of his influence he had never radiated before.

Hume was radiating attar of roses.

II

On Thursday night Horace Tarbox sat in an aisle seat in the fifth row and witnessed "Home James." Oddly enough he found that he was enjoying himself. The cynical students near him were annoyed at his audible appreciation of time-honoured jokes in the Hammerstein tradition. But Horace was waiting with anxiety for Marcia Meadow singing her song about a Jazz-bound Blundering Blimp. When she did appear, radiant under a floppity flower-faced hat, a warm glow settled over him, and when the song was over he did not join in the storm of applause. He felt somewhat numb.

In the intermission after the second act an usher materialized beside him, demanded to know if he were Mr. Tarbox, and then handed him a note written in a round adolescent band. Horace read it in some confusion, while the usher lingered with withering patience in the aisle.

> "Dear Omar:
>
> *After the show I always grow an awful hunger.*
> *If you want to satisfy it for me in the Taft Grill*
> *just communicate your answer to the big-timber guide*
> *that brought this and oblige.*
>   *Your friend,*
>   *Marcia Meadow."*

"Tell her,"—he coughed—"tell her that it will be quite all right. I'll meet her in front of the theatre."

The big-timber guide smiled arrogantly.

"I giss she meant for you to come roun' t' the stage door."

"Where—where is it?"

"Ou'side. Tunayulef. Down ee alley."

"What?"

"Ou'side. Turn to y' left! Down ee alley!"

The arrogant person withdrew. A freshman behind Horace snickered.

Then half an hour later, sitting in the Taft Grill opposite the hair that was yellow by natural pigment, the prodigy was saying an odd thing.

"Do you have to do that dance in the last act?" he was asking earnestly—"I mean, would they dismiss you if you refused to do it?"

Marcia grinned.

"It's fun to do it. I like to do it."

And then Horace came out with a faux pas.

"I should think you'd detest it," he remarked succinctly. "The people behind me were making remarks about your bosom."

Marcia blushed fiery red.

"I can't help that," she said quickly. "The dance to me is only a sort of acrobatic stunt. Lord, it's hard enough to do! I rub liniment into my shoulders for an hour every night."

"Do you have—fun while you're on the stage?"

"Uh-huh—sure! I got in the habit of having people look at me, Omar, and I like it."

"Hm!" Horace sank into a brownish study.

"How's the Brazilian trimmings?"

"Hm!" repeated Horace, and then after a pause: "Where does the play go from here?"

"New York."

"For how long?"

"All depends. Winter—maybe."

"Oh!"

"Coming up to lay eyes on me, Omar, or aren't you int'rested? Not as nice here, is it, as it was up in your room? I wish we was there now."

"I feel idiotic in this place," confessed Horace, looking round him nervously.

"Too bad! We got along pretty well."

At this he looked suddenly so melancholy that she changed her tone, and reaching over patted his hand.

"Ever take an actress out to supper before?"

"No," said Horace miserably, "and I never will again. I don't know why I came to-night. Here under all these lights and with all these people laughing and chattering I feel completely out of my sphere. I don't know what to talk to you about."

"We'll talk about me. We talked about you last time."

"Very well."

"Well, my name really is Meadow, but my first name isn't Marcia—it's Veronica. I'm nineteen. Question—how did the girl make her leap to the footlights? Answer—she was born in Passaic, New Jersey, and up to a year ago she got the right to breathe by pushing Nabiscoes in Marcel's tea-room in Trenton. She started going with a guy named Robbins, a singer in the Trent House cabaret, and he got her to try a song and dance with him one evening. In a month we were filling the supperroom every night. Then we went to New York with meet-my-friend letters thick as a pile of napkins.

"In two days we landed a job at Divinerries', and I learned to shimmy from a kid at the Palais Royal. We stayed at Divinerries' six months until one night Peter Boyce Wendell, the columnist, ate his milk-toast there. Next morning a poem about Marvellous Marcia came out in his newspaper, and within two days I had three vaudeville offers and a chance at the Midnight Frolic. I wrote Wendell a thank you letter, and he printed it in his column—said that the style was like Carlyle's, only more rugged and that I ought to quit dancing and do North American literature. This got me a coupla more vaudeville offers and a chance as an *ingénue* in a regular show. I took it—and here I am, Omar."

When she finished they sat for a moment in silence she draping the last skeins of a Welsh rabbit on her fork and waiting for him to speak.

"Let's get out of here," he said suddenly.

Marcia's eyes hardened.

"What's the idea? Am I making you sick?"

"No, but I don't like it here. I don't like to be sitting here with you."

Without another word Marcia signalled for the waiter.

"What's the check?" she demanded briskly "My part—the rabbit and the ginger ale."

Horace watched blankly as the waiter figured it.

"See here," he began, "I intended to pay for yours too. You're my guest."

With a half-sigh Marcia rose from the table and walked from the room. Horace, his face a document in bewilderment, laid a bill down and followed her out, up the stairs and into the lobby. He overtook her in front of the elevator and they faced each other.

"See here," he repeated "You're my guest. Have I said something to offend you?"

After an instant of wonder Marcia's eyes softened.

"You're a rude fella!" she said slowly. "Don't you know you're rude?"

"I can't help it," said Horace with a directness she found quite disarming. "You know I like you."

"You said you didn't like being with me."

"I didn't like it."

"Why not?" Fire blazed suddenly from the grey forests of his eyes.

"Because I didn't. I've formed the habit of liking you. I've been thinking of nothing much else for two days."

"Well, if you—"

"Wait a minute," he interrupted. "I've got something to say. It's this: in six weeks I'll be eighteen years old. When I'm eighteen years old I'm coming up to New York to see you. Is there some place in New York where we can go and not have a lot of people in the room?"

"Sure!" smiled Marcia. "You can come up to my 'partment. Sleep on the couch if you want to."

"I can't sleep on couches," he said shortly. "But I want to talk to you."

"Why, sure," repeated Marcia. "in my 'partment."

In his excitement Horace put his hands in his pockets.

"All right—just so I can see you alone. I want to talk to you as we talked up in my room."

"Honey boy," cried Marcia, laughing, "is it that you want to kiss me?"

"Yes," Horace almost shouted. "I'll kiss you if you want me to."

The elevator man was looking at them reproachfully. Marcia edged toward the grated door.

"I'll drop you a postcard," she said.

Horace's eyes were quite wild.

"Send me a postcard! I'll come up any time after January first. I'll be eighteen then."

And as she stepped into the elevator he coughed enigmatically, yet with a vague challenge, at the calling, and walked quickly away.

III

He was there again. She saw him when she took her first glance at the restless Manhattan audience—down in the front row with his head bent a bit forward and his grey eyes fixed on her. And she knew that to him they were alone together in a world where the high-rouged row of ballet faces and the massed whines of the violins were as imperceivable as powder on a marble Venus. An instinctive defiance rose within her.

"Silly boy!" she said to herself hurriedly, and she didn't take her encore.

"What do they expect for a hundred a week—perpetual motion?" she grumbled to herself in the wings.

"What's the trouble? Marcia?"

"Guy I don't like down in front."

During the last act as she waited for her specialty she had an odd attack of stage fright. She had never sent Horace the promised post-card. Last night she had pretended not to see him—had hurried from the theatre immediately after her dance to pass a sleepless night in her apartment, thinking—as she had so often in the last month—of his pale, rather intent face, his slim, boyish figure, the merciless, unworldly abstraction that made him charming to her.

And now that he had come she felt vaguely sorry—as though an unwonted responsibility was being forced on her.

"Infant prodigy!" she said aloud.

"What?" demanded the negro comedian standing beside her.

"Nothing—just talking about myself."

On the stage she felt better. This was her dance—and she always felt that the way she did it wasn't suggestive any more than to some men every pretty girl is suggestive. She made it a stunt.

> *"Uptown, downtown, jelly on a spoon,*
> *After sundown shiver by the moon."*

He was not watching her now. She saw that clearly. He was looking very deliberately at a castle on the back drop, wearing that expression he had worn in the Taft Grill. A wave of exasperation swept over her—he was criticising her.

> *"That's the vibration that thrills me,*
> *Funny how affection fi-lls me*
> *Uptown, downtown—"*

Unconquerable revulsion seized her. She was suddenly and horribly conscious of her audience as she had never been since her first appearance. Was that a leer on a pallid face in the front row, a droop of disgust on one young girl's mouth? These shoulders of hers—these shoulders shaking—were they hers? Were they real? Surely shoulders weren't made for this!

> *"Then—you'll see at a glance*
> *"I'll need some funeral ushers with St. Vitus dance*
> *At the end of the world I'll—"*

The bassoon and two cellos crashed into a final chord. She paused and poised a moment on her toes with every muscle tense, her young face looking out dully at the audience in what one young girl afterward called "such a curious, puzzled look," and then without bowing rushed from the stage. Into the dressing-room she sped, kicked out of one dress and into another, and caught a taxi outside.

Her apartment was very warm—small, it was, with a row of professional pictures and sets of Kipling and O. Henry which she had bought once from a blue-eyed agent and read occasionally. And there were several chairs which matched, but were none of them comfortable, and a pink-shaded lamp with blackbirds painted on it and an atmosphere of other stifled pink throughout. There were nice things in it—nice things unrelentingly hostile to each other, offspring of a vicarious, impatient taste acting in stray moments. The worst was typified by a great picture framed in oak bark of Passaic as seen from the Erie Railroad—altogether a frantic, oddly extravagant, oddly penurious attempt to make a cheerful room. Marcia knew it was a failure.

Into this room came the prodigy and took her two hands awkwardly.

"I followed you this time," he said.

"Oh!"

"I want you to marry me," he said.

Her arms went out to him. She kissed his mouth with a sort of passionate wholesomeness.

"There!"

"I love you," he said.

She kissed him again and then with a little sigh flung herself into an armchair and half lay there, shaken with absurd laughter.

"Why, you infant prodigy!" she cried.

"Very well, call me that if you want to. I once told you that I was ten thousand years older than you—I am."

She laughed again.

"I don't like to be disapproved of."

"No one's ever going to disapprove of you again."

"Omar," she asked, "why do you want to marry me?"

The prodigy rose and put his hands in his pockets.

"Because I love you, Marcia Meadow."

And then she stopped calling him Omar.

"Dear boy," she said, "you know I sort of love you. There's something about you—I can't tell what—that just puts my heart through the wringer every time I'm round you. But honey—" She paused.

"But what?"

"But lots of things. But you're only just eighteen, and I'm nearly twenty."

"Nonsense!" he interrupted. "Put it this way—that I'm in my nineteenth year and you're nineteen. That makes us pretty close—without counting that other ten thousand years I mentioned."

Marcia laughed.

"But there are some more 'buts.' Your people—"

"My people!" exclaimed the prodigy ferociously. "My people tried to make a monstrosity out of me." His face grew quite crimson at the enormity of what he was going to say. "My people can go way back and sit down!"

"My heavens!" cried Marcia in alarm. "All that? On tacks, I suppose."

"Tacks—yes," he agreed wildly—"on anything. The more I think of how they allowed me to become a little dried-up mummy—"

"What makes you think you're that?" asked Marcia quietly—"me?"

"Yes. Every person I've met on the streets since I met you has made me jealous because they knew what love was before I did. I used to call it the 'sex impulse.' Heavens!"

"There's more 'buts,'" said Marcia

"What are they?"

"How could we live?"

"I'll make a living."

"You're in college."

"Do you think I care anything about taking a Master of Arts degree?"

"You want to be Master of Me, hey?"

"Yes! What? I mean, no!"

Marcia laughed, and crossing swiftly over sat in his lap. He put his arm round her wildly and implanted the vestige of a kiss somewhere near her neck.

"There's something white about you," mused Marcia "but it doesn't sound very logical."

"Oh, don't be so darned reasonable!"

"I can't help it," said Marcia.

"I hate these slot-machine people!"

"But we—"

"Oh, shut up!"

And as Marcia couldn't talk through her ears she had to.

IV

Horace and Marcia were married early in February. The sensation in academic circles both at Yale and Princeton was tremendous. Horace Tarbox, who at fourteen had been played up in the Sunday magazines sections of metropolitan newspapers, was throwing over his career, his chance of being a world authority on American philosophy, by marrying a chorus girl—they made Marcia a chorus girl. But like all modern stories it was a four-and-a-half-day wonder.

They took a flat in Harlem. After two weeks' search,

during which his idea of the value of academic knowledge faded unmercifully, Horace took a position as clerk with a South American export company—someone had told him that exporting was the coming thing. Marcia was to stay in her show for a few months anyway until he got on his feet. He was getting a hundred and twenty-five to start with, and though of course they told him it was only a question of months until he would be earning double that, Marcia refused even to consider giving up the hundred and fifty a week that she was getting at the time.

"We'll call ourselves Head and Shoulders, dear," she said softly, "and the shoulders'll have to keep shaking a little longer until the old head gets started."

"I hate it," he objected gloomily.

"Well," she replied emphatically, "Your salary wouldn't keep us in a tenement. Don't think I want to be public—I don't. I want to be yours. But I'd be a half-wit to sit in one room and count the sunflowers on the wall-paper while I waited for you. When you pull down three hundred a month I'll quit."

And much as it hurt his pride, Horace had to admit that hers was the wiser course.

March mellowed into April. May read a gorgeous riot act to the parks and waters of Manhattan, and they were very happy. Horace, who had no habits whatsoever—he had never had time to form any—proved the most adaptable of husbands, and as Marcia entirely lacked opinions on the subjects that engrossed him there were very few jottings and bumpings. Their minds moved in different spheres. Marcia acted as practical factotum, and Horace lived either in his old world of abstract ideas or in a sort of triumphantly earthy worship and adoration of his wife. She was a continual source of astonishment to him—the freshness and originality of her mind, her dynamic, clear-headed energy, and her unfailing good humour.

And Marcia's co-workers in the nine-o'clock show, whither she had transferred her talents, were impressed with her tremendous pride in her husband's mental powers. Horace they knew only as a very slim, tight-lipped, and immature-looking young man, who waited every night to take her home.

"Horace," said Marcia one evening when she met him as usual at eleven, "you looked like a ghost standing there against the street lights. You losing weight?"

He shook his head vaguely.

"I don't know. They raised me to a hundred and thirty-five dollars to-day, and—"

"I don't care," said Marcia severely. "You're killing yourself working at night. You read those big books on economy—"

"Economics," corrected Horace.

"Well, you read 'em every night long after I'm asleep. And you're getting all stooped over like you were before we were married."

"But, Marcia, I've got to—"

"No, you haven't dear. I guess I'm running this shop for the present, and I won't let my fella ruin his health and eyes. You got to get some exercise."

"I do. Every morning I—"

"Oh, I know! But those dumb-bells of yours wouldn't give a consumptive two degrees of fever. I mean real exercise. You've got to join a gymnasium. 'Member you told me you were such a trick gymnast once that they tried to get you out for the team in college and they couldn't because you had a standing date with Herb Spencer?"

"I used to enjoy it," mused Horace, "but it would take up too much time now."

"All right," said Marcia. "I'll make a bargain with you. You join a gym and I'll read one of those books from the brown row of 'em."

"'Pepys' Diary'? Why, that ought to be enjoyable. He's very light."

"Not for me—he isn't. It'll be like digesting plate glass. But you been telling me how much it'd broaden my lookout. Well, you go to a gym three nights a week and I'll take one big dose of Sammy."

Horace hesitated.

"Well—"

"Come on, now! You do some giant swings for me and I'll chase some culture for you."

So Horace finally consented, and all through a baking summer he spent three and sometimes four evenings a week experimenting on the trapeze in Skipper's Gymnasium. And in August he admitted to Marcia that it made him capable of more mental work during the day.

"*Mens sana in corpore sano,*" he said.

"Don't believe in it," replied Marcia. "I tried one of those patent medicines once and they're all bunk. You stick to gymnastics."

One night in early September while he was going through one of his contortions on the rings in the nearly deserted room he was addressed by a meditative fat man whom he had noticed watching him for several nights.

"Say, lad, do that stunt you were doin' last night."

Horace grinned at him from his perch.

"I invented it," he said. "I got the idea from the fourth proposition of Euclid."

"What circus he with?"

"He's dead."

"Well, he must of broke his neck doin' that stunt. I set here last night thinkin' sure you was goin' to break yours."

"Like this!" said Horace, and swinging onto the trapeze he did his stunt.

"Don't it kill your neck an' shoulder muscles?"

"It did at first, but inside of a week I wrote the quod eras demonstrandum on it."

"Hm!"

Horace swung idly on the trapeze.

"Ever think of takin' it up professionally?" asked the fat man.

"Not I."

"Good money in it if you're willin' to do stunts like 'at an' can get away with it."

"Here's another," chirped Horace eagerly, and the fat man's mouth dropped suddenly agape as he watched this pink-jerseyed Prometheus again defy the gods and Isaac Newton.

The night following this encounter Horace got home from work to find a rather pale Marcia stretched out on the sofa waiting for him.

"I fainted twice to-day," she began without preliminaries.

"What?"

"Yep. You see baby's due in four months now. Doctor says I ought to have quit dancing two weeks ago."

Horace sat down and thought it over.

"I'm glad of course," he said pensively—"I mean glad that we're going to have a baby. But this means a lot of expense."

"I've got two hundred and fifty in the bank," said Marcia hopefully, "and two weeks' pay coming."

Horace computed quickly.

"Including my salary, that'll give us nearly fourteen hundred for the next six months."

Marcia looked blue.

"That all? Course I can get a job singing somewhere this month. And I can go to work again in March."

"Of course nothing!" said Horace gruffly. "You'll stay right here. Let's see now—there'll be doctor's bills and a nurse, besides the maid: We've got to have some more money."

"Well," said Marcia wearily, "I don't know where it's coming from. It's up to the old head now. Shoulders is out of business."

Horace rose and pulled on his coat.

"Where are you going?"

"I've got an idea," he answered. "I'll be right back."

Ten minutes later as he headed down the street toward Skipper's Gymnasium he felt a placid wonder, quite unmixed with humour, at what he was going to do. How he would have gaped at himself a year before! How everyone would have gaped! But when you opened your door at the rap of life you let in many things.

The gymnasium was brightly lit, and when his eyes became accustomed to the glare he found the meditative fat man seated on a pile of canvas mats smoking a big cigar.

"Say," began Horace directly, "were you in earnest last night when you said I could make money on my trapeze stunts?"

"Why, yes," said the fat man in surprise.

"Well, I've been thinking it over, and I believe I'd like to try it. I could work at night and on Saturday afternoons—and regularly if the pay is high enough."

The fat man looked at his watch.

"Well," he said, "Charlie Paulson's the man to see. He'll book you inside of four days, once he sees you work out. He won't be in now, but I'll get hold of him for to-morrow night."

The fat man was as good as his word. Charlie Paulson arrived next night and put in a wondrous hour watching the prodigy swoop through the air in amazing parabolas, and on the night following he brought two large men with him who looked as though they had been born smoking black cigars and talking about money in low, passionate voices. Then on the succeeding Saturday Horace Tarbox's torso made its first professional appearance in a gymnastic exhibition at the Coleman Street Gardens. But though the audience numbered nearly five thousand people, Horace felt no nervousness. From his childhood he had read papers to audiences—learned that trick of detaching himself.

"Marcia," he said cheerfully later that same night, "I think we're out of the woods. Paulson thinks he can get me an opening at the Hippodrome, and that means an all-winter engagement. The Hippodrome you know, is a big—"

"Yes, I believe I've heard of it," interrupted Marcia, "but I want to know about this stunt you're doing. It isn't any spectacular suicide, is it?"

"It's nothing," said Horace quietly. "But if you can think of a nicer way of a man killing himself than taking a risk for you, why that's the way I want to die."

Marcia reached up and wound both arms tightly round his neck.

"Kiss me," she whispered, "and call me 'dear heart.' I love to hear you say 'dear heart.' And bring me a book to read to-morrow. No more Sam Pepys, but something trick and trashy. I've been wild for something to do all day. I felt like writing letters, but I didn't have anybody to write to."

"Write to me," said Horace. "I'll read them."

"I wish I could," breathed Marcia. "If I knew words enough I could write you the longest love-letter in the world—and never get tired."

But after two more months Marcia grew very tired indeed, and for a row of nights it was a very anxious, weary-looking young athlete who walked out before the Hippodrome crowd. Then there were two days when his place was taken by a young man who wore pale blue instead of white, and got very little applause. But after the two days Horace appeared again, and those who sat close to the stage remarked an expression of beatific happiness on that young acrobat's face even when he was twisting breathlessly in the air in the middle of his amazing and original shoulder swing. After that performance he laughed at the elevator man and dashed up the stairs to the flat five steps at a time—and then tiptoed very carefully into a quiet room.

"Marcia," he whispered.

"Hello!" She smiled up at him wanly. "Horace, there's something I want you to do. Look in my top bureau drawer and you'll find a big stack of paper. It's a book—sort of—Horace. I wrote it down in these last three months while I've been laid up. I wish you'd take it to that Peter Boyce Wendell who put my letter in his paper. He could tell you whether it'd be a good book. I wrote it just the way I talk, just the way I wrote that letter to him. It's just a story about a lot of things that happened to me. Will you take it to him, Horace?"

"Yes, darling."

He leaned over the bed until his head was beside her on the pillow, and began stroking back her yellow hair.

"Dearest Marcia," he said softly.

"No," she murmured, "call me what I told you to call me."

"Dear heart," he whispered passionately—"dearest heart."

"What'll we call her?"

They rested a minute in happy, drowsy content, while Horace considered.

"We'll call her Marcia Hume Tarbox," he said at length.

"Why the Hume?"

"Because he's the fellow who first introduced us."

"That so?" she murmured, sleepily surprised. "I thought his name was Moon."

Her eyes closed, and after a moment the slow lengthening surge of the bedclothes over her breast showed that she was asleep.

Horace tiptoed over to the bureau and opening the top drawer found a heap of closely scrawled, lead-smeared pages. He looked at the first sheet:

SANDRA PEPYS, SYNCOPATED
BY MARCIA TARBOX

He smiled. So Samuel Pepys had made an impression on her after all. He turned a page and began to read. His smile deepened—he read on. Half an hour passed and he became aware that Marcia had waked and was watching him from the bed.

"Honey," came in a whisper.

"What Marcia?"

"Do you like it?"

Horace coughed.

"I seem to be reading on. It's bright."

"Take it to Peter Boyce Wendell. Tell him you got the

highest marks in Princeton once and that you ought to know when a book's good. Tell him this one's a world beater."

"All right, Marcia," Horace said gently.

Her eyes closed again and Horace crossing over kissed her forehead—stood there for a moment with a look of tender pity. Then he left the room.

All that night the sprawly writing on the pages, the constant mistakes in spelling and grammar, and the weird punctuation danced before his eyes. He woke several times in the night, each time full of a welling chaotic sympathy for this desire of Marcia's soul to express itself in words. To him there was something infinitely pathetic about it, and for the first time in months he began to turn over in his mind his own half-forgotten dreams.

He had meant to write a series of books, to popularise the new realism as Schopenhauer had popularised pessimism and William James pragmatism.

But life hadn't come that way. Life took hold of people and forced them into flying rings. He laughed to think of that rap at his door, the diaphanous shadow in Hume, Marcia's threatened kiss.

"And it's still me," he said aloud in wonder as he lay awake in the darkness. "I'm the man who sat in Berkeley with temerity to wonder if that rap would have had actual existence had my ear not been there to hear it. I'm still that man. I could be electrocuted for the crimes he committed.

"Poor gauzy souls trying to express ourselves in something tangible. Marcia with her written book; I with my unwritten ones. Trying to choose our mediums and then taking what we get—and being glad."

V

"Sandra Pepys, Syncopated," with an introduction by Peter Boyce Wendell the columnist, appeared serially in Jordan's Magazine, and came out in book form in March. From its first published instalment it attracted attention far and wide. A trite enough subject—a girl from a small New Jersey town coming to New York to go on the stage—treated simply, with a peculiar vividness of phrasing and a haunting undertone of sadness in the very inadequacy of its vocabulary, it made an irresistible appeal.

Peter Boyce Wendell, who happened at that time to be advocating the enrichment of the American language by the immediate adoption of expressive vernacular words, stood as its sponsor and thundered his indorsement over the placid bromides of the conventional reviewers.

Marcia received three hundred dollars an instalment for the serial publication, which came at an opportune time, for though Horace's monthly salary at the Hippodrome was now more than Marcia's had ever been, young Marcia was emitting shrill cries which they intepreted as a demand for country air. So early April found them installed in a bungalow in Westchester County, with a place for a lawn, a place for a garage, and a place for everything, including a sound-proof impregnable study, in which Marcia faithfully promised Mr. Jordan she would shut herself up when her daughter's demands began to be abated, and compose immortally illiterate literature.

"It's not half bad," thought Horace one night as he was on his way from the station to his house. He was considering several prospects that had opened up, a four months' vaudeville offer in five figures, a chance to go back to Princeton in charge of all gymnasium work. Odd! He had once intended to go back there in charge of all philosophic work, and now he had not even been stirred by the arrival in New York of Anton Laurier, his old idol.

The gravel crunched raucously under his heel. He saw the lights of his sitting-room gleaming and noticed a big car standing in the drive. Probably Mr. Jordan again, come to persuade Marcia to settle down to work.

She had heard the sound of his approach and her form was silhouetted against the lighted door as she came out to meet him.

"There's some Frenchman here," she whispered nervously. "I can't pronounce his name, but he sounds awful deep. You'll have to jaw with him."

"What Frenchman?"

"You can't prove it by me. He drove up an hour ago with Mr. Jordan, and said he wanted to meet Sandra Pepys, and all that sort of thing."

Two men rose from chairs as they went inside.

"Hello Tarbox," said Jordan. "I've just been bringing together two celebrities. I've brought M'sieur Laurier out with me. M'sieur Laurier, let me present Mr. Tarbox, Mrs. Tarbox s husband."

"Not Anton Laurier!" exclaimed Horace.

"But, yes. I must come. I have to come. I have read the book of Madame, and I have been charmed"—he fumbled in his pocket—"ah I have read of you too. In this newspaper which I read to-day it has your name."

He finally produced a clipping from a magazine.

"Read it!" he said eagerly. "It has about you too."

Horace's eye skipped down the page.

"A distinct contribution to American dialect literature," it said. "No attempt at literary tone; the book derives its very quality from this fact, as did 'Huckle-berry Finn.'"

Horace's eyes caught a passage lower down; he became suddenly aghast—read on hurriedly:

"Marcia Tarbox's connection with the stage is not only as a spectator but as the wife of a performer. She was married last year to Horace Tarbox, who every evening delights the children at the Hippodrome with his wondrous flying performance. It is said that the young couple have dubbed themselves Head and Shoulders, referring doubtless to the fact that Mrs. Tarbox supplies the literary and mental qualities, while the supple and agile shoulders of her husband contribute their share to the family fortunes.

"Mrs. Tarbox seems to merit that much-abused title—'prodigy.' Only twenty—"

Horace stopped reading, and with a very odd expression in his eyes gazed intently at Anton Laurier.

"I want to advise you—" he began hoarsely.

"What?"

"About raps. Don't answer them! Let them alone—have a padded door."

Harriet Beecher Stowe

A Scholar's Adventures in the Country

"If we could only live in the country," said my wife, "how much easier it would be to live!"

"And how much cheaper!" said I.

"To have a little place of our own, and raise our own things!" said my wife. "Dear me! I am heartsick when I think of the old place at home, and father's great garden. What peaches and melons we used to have! what green peas and corn! Now one has to buy every cent's worth of these things—and how they taste! Such wilted, miserable corn! Such peas! Then, if we lived in the country, we should have our own cow, and milk and cream in abundance; our own hens and chickens. We could have custard and ice-cream every day."

"To say nothing of the trees and flowers, and all that," said I.

The result of this little domestic duet was that my wife and I began to ride about the city of —— to look up some pretty, interesting cottage, where our visions of rural bliss might be realized. Country residences, near the city, we found to bear rather a high price; so that it was no easy matter to find a situation suitable to the length of our purse; till, at last, a judicious friend suggested a happy expedient.

"Borrow a few hundred," he said, "and give your note; you can save enough, very soon, to make the difference. When you raise everything you eat, you know it will make your salary go a wonderful deal further."

"Certainly it will," said I. "And what can be more beautiful than to buy places by the simple process of giving one's note?—'tis so neat, and handy, and convenient!"

"Why," pursued my friend, "there is Mr. B., my next-door neighbour—'tis enough to make one sick of life in the city to spend a week out on his farm. Such princely living as one gets! And he assures me that it costs him very little—scarce anything perceptible, in fact."

"Indeed!" said I; "few people can say that."

"Why," said my friend, "he has a couple of peach-trees for every month, from June till frost, that furnish as many peaches as he, and his wife, and ten children can dispose of. And then he has grapes, apricots, etc.; and last year his wife sold fifty dollars worth from her strawberry patch, and had an abundance for the table besides. Out of the milk of only one cow they had butter enough to sell three or four pounds a week, besides abundance of milk and cream; and madam has the butter for her pocket money. This is the way country people manage."

"Glorious!" thought I. And my wife and I could scarcely sleep, all night, for the brilliancy of our anticipations!

To be sure our delight was somewhat damped the next day by the coldness with which my good old uncle, Jeremiah Standfast, who happened along at precisely this crisis, listened to our visions.

"You'll find it pleasant, children, in the summer time," said the hard-fisted old man, twirling his blue-checked pocket-handkerchief; "but I'm sorry you've gone in debt for the land."

"Oh, but we shall soon save that—it's so much cheaper living in the country!" said both of us together.

"Well, as to that, I don't think it is, to city-bred folks."

Here I broke in with a flood of accounts of Mr. B.'s peach-trees, and Mrs. B.'s strawberries, butter, apricots, etc., etc.; to which the old gentleman listened with such a long, leathery, unmoved quietude of visage as quite provoked me, and gave me the worst possible opinion of his judgment. I was disappointed, too; for as he was reckoned one of the best practical farmers in the county, I had counted on an enthusiastic sympathy with all my agricultural designs.

"I tell you what, children," he said, "a body can live in the country, as you say, amazin' cheap; but then a body must *know how*,"—and my uncle spread his pocket-handkerchief thoughtfully out upon his knees, and shook his head gravely.

I thought him a terribly slow, stupid old body, and wondered how I had always entertained so high an opinion of his sense.

"He is evidently getting old," said I to my wife; "his judgment is not what it used to be."

At all events, our place was bought, and we moved out, well pleased, the first morning in April, not at all remembering the ill savour of that day for matters of wisdom. Our place was a pretty cottage, about two miles from the city, with grounds that had been tastefully laid out. There was no lack of winding paths, arbours, flower borders, and rosebushes, with which my wife was especially pleased. There was a little green lot, strolling off down to a brook, with a thick grove of trees at the end, where our cow was to be pastured.

The first week or two went on happily enough in getting our little new pet of a house into trimness and good order; for as it had been long for sale, of course there was any amount of little repairs that had been left to amuse the leisure hours of the purchaser. Here a doorstep had given way, and needed replacing; there a shutter hung loose, and wanted a hinge; abundance of glass needed setting; and as to painting and papering, there was no end to that. Then my wife wanted a door cut here, to make our bedroom more convenient, and a china closet knocked up there, where no china closet before had been. We even ventured on throwing out a bay-window from our sitting-room, because we had luckily lighted on a workman who was so cheap that it was an actual saving of money to employ him. And to be sure our darling little cottage did lift up its head wonderfully for all this garnishing and furbishing. I got up early every morning, and nailed up the rosebushes, and my wife got up and watered geraniums, and both flattered ourselves and each other on our early hours and thrifty habits. But soon, like Adam and Eve in Paradise, we found our little domain to ask more hands than ours to get it into shape. So says I to my wife, "I will bring out a gardener when I come next time, and he shall lay the garden out, and get it into order; and after that I can easily keep it by the work of my leisure hours."

Our gardener was a very sublime sort of man,—an Englishman, and of course used to laying out noblemen's places,—and we became as grasshoppers in our own eyes when he talked of Lord This and That's estate, and began to question us about our carriage drive and conservatory; and we could with difficulty bring the gentleman down to any understanding of the humble limits of our expectations; merely to dress out the walks, and lay out a kitchen garden, and plant potatoes, turnips, beets and carrots, was quite a descent for him. In fact, so strong were his aesthetic preferences, that he persuaded my wife to let him dig all the turf off from a green square opposite the bay window, and to lay it out into divers little triangles, resembling small pieces of pie, together with circles, mounds, and various other geometrical ornaments, the planning and planting of which soon engrossed my wife's whole soul. The planting of the potatoes, beets, carrots, etc., was intrusted to a raw Irishman; for as to me, to confess the truth, I began to fear that digging did not agree with me. It is true that I was exceedingly vigorous at first, and actually planted with my own hands two or three long rows of potatoes; after which I got a turn of rheumatism in my shoulder, which lasted me a week. Stooping down to plant beets and radishes gave me a vertigo, so that I was obliged to content myself with a general superintendence of the garden; that is to say, I charged my Englishman to see that my Irishman did his duty properly, and then got on to my horse and rode to the city. But about one part of the matter, I must say, I was not remiss; and that is, in the purchase of seed and garden utensils. Not a day passed that I did not come home with my pockets stuffed with choice seeds, roots, etc.; and the variety of my garden utensils was unequalled. There was not a priming hook of any pattern, not a hoe, rake, or spade great or small, that I did not have specimens of; and flower seeds and bulbs were also forthcoming in liberal proportions. In fact, I had opened an account at a thriving seed store; for when a man is driving business on a large scale, it is not always convenient to hand out the change for every little matter, and buying things on account is as neat and agreeable a mode of acquisition as paying bills with one's notes.

"You know we must have a cow," said my wife, the

morning of our second week. Our friend the gardener, who had now worked with us at the rate of two dollars a day for two weeks, was at hand in a moment in our emergency. We wanted to buy a cow, and he had one to sell—a wonderful cow, of a real English breed. He would not sell her for any money, except to oblige particular friends; but as we had patronized him, we should have her for forty dollars. How much we were obliged to him! The forty dollars were speedily forthcoming, and so also was the cow.

"What makes her shake her head in that way?" said my wife, apprehensively, as she observed the interesting beast making sundry demonstrations with her horns. "I hope she's gentle."

The gardener fluently demonstrated that the animal was a pattern of all the softer graces, and that this head-shaking was merely a little nervous affection consequent on the embarrassment of a new position. We had faith to believe almost anything at this time, and therefore came from the barn yard to the house as much satisfied with our purchase as Job with his three thousand camels and five hundred yoke of oxen. Her quondam master milked her for us the first evening, out of a delicate regard to her feelings as a stranger, and we fancied that we discerned forty dollars' worth of excellence in the very quality of the milk.

But alas! the next morning our Irish girl came in with a most rueful face. "And is it milking that baste you'd have me be after?" she said; "sure, and she won't let me come near her."

"Nonsense, Biddy!" said I; "you frightened her, perhaps; the cow is perfectly gentle;" and with the pail on my arm I sallied forth. The moment madam saw me entering the cow yard, she greeted me with a very expressive flourish of her horns.

"This won't do," said I, and I stopped. The lady evidently was serious in her intentions of resisting any personal approaches. I cut a cudgel, and, putting on a bold face, marched towards her, while Biddy followed with her milking stool. Apparently the beast saw the necessity of temporizing, for she assumed a demure expression, and Biddy sat down to milk. I stood sentry, and if the lady shook her head I shook my stick; and thus the milking operation proceeded with tolerable serenity and success.

"There!" said I, with dignity, when the frothing pail was full to the brim. "That will do, Biddy," and I dropped my stick. Dump! came madam's heel on the side of the pail, and it flew like a rocket into the air, while the milky flood showered plentifully over me, and a new broadcloth riding-coat that I had assumed for the first time that morning. "Whew!" said I, as soon as I could get my breath from this extraordinary shower bath; "what's all this?" My wife came running towards the cow yard, as I stood with the milk streaming from my hair, filling my eyes, and dropping from the tip of my nose; and she and Biddy performed a recitative lamentation over me in alternate strophes, like the chorus in a Greek tragedy. Such was our first morning's experience; but as we had announced our bargain with some considerable flourish of trumpets among our neighbours and friends, we concluded to hush the matter up as much as possible.

"These very superior cows are apt to be cross," said I; "we must bear with it as we do with the eccentricities of genius; besides, when she gets accustomed to us, it will be better."

Madam was therefore installed into her pretty pasture lot, and my wife contemplated with pleasure the picturesque effect of her appearance, reclining on the green slope of the pasture lot, or standing ankle deep in the gurgling brook, or reclining under the deep shadows of the trees. She was, in fact, a handsome cow, which may account, in part, for some of her sins; and this consideration inspired me with some degree of indulgence towards her foibles.

But when I found that Biddy could never succeed in getting near her in the pasture, and that any kind of success in the milking operations required my vigorous personal exertions morning and evening, the matter wore a more serious aspect, and I began to feel quite pensive and apprehensive. It is very well to talk of the pleasures of the milkmaid going out in the balmy freshness of the purple dawn; but imagine a poor fellow pulled out of bed on a drizzly, rainy morning, and equipping himself for a scamper through a wet pasture lot, rope in hand, at the heels of such a termagant as mine! In fact, madam established a regular series of exercises, which had all to be gone through before she would suffer herself to be captured; as, first, she would station herself plump in the middle of a marsh, which lay at the lower part of the lot, and look very innocent and absent-minded, as if reflecting on some sentimental subject. "Suke! Suke! Suke!" I ejaculate, cautiously tottering along the edge of the marsh, and holding out an ear of corn. The lady looks gracious, and comes forward, almost within reach of my hand. I make a plunge to throw the rope over her horns, and away she goes, kicking up mud and water into my face in her flight, while I, losing my balance, tumble forward into the marsh. I pick myself up, and, full of wrath, behold her placidly chewing her cud on the other side, with the meekest air imaginable, as who should say, "I hope you are not hurt, sir." I dash through swamp and bog furiously, resolving to carry all by a coup de main. Then follows a miscellaneous season of dodging, scampering, and bopeeping, among the trees of the grove, interspersed with sundry occasional races across the bog aforesaid. I always wondered how I caught her every day; and when I had tied her head to one post and her heels to another, I wiped the sweat from my brow, and thought I was paying dear for the eccentricities of genius. A genius she certainly was, for besides her surprising agility, she had other talents equally extraordinary. There was no fence that she could not take down; nowhere that she could not go. She took the pickets off the garden fence at her pleasure, using her horns as handily as I could use a claw hammer. Whatever she had a mind to, whether it were a bite in the cabbage garden, or a run in the corn patch, or a foraging expedition into the flower borders, she made herself equally welcome and at home. Such a scampering and driving, such cries of "Suke here" and "Suke there," as constantly greeted our ears, kept our little establishment in a constant commotion. At last, when she one morning made a plunge at the skirts of my new broadcloth frock coat, and carried off one flap on her horns, my patience gave out, and I determined to sell her.

As, however, I had made a good story of my misfortunes among my friends and neighbours, and amused them with sundry whimsical accounts of my various adventures in the cow-catching line, I found, when I came to speak of selling, that there was a general coolness on the subject, and nobody seemed disposed to be the recipient of my responsibilities. In short, I was glad, at last, to get fifteen dollars for her, and comforted myself with thinking that I had at least gained twenty-five dollars worth of experience in the transaction, to say nothing of the fine exercise.

I comforted my soul, however, the day after, by purchasing and bringing home to my wife a fine swarm of bees.

"Your bee, now," says I, "is a really classical insect, and breathes of Virgil and the Augustan age,—and then she is a domestic, tranquil, placid creature. How beautiful the murmuring of a hive near our honeysuckle of a calm, summer evening! Then they are tranquilly and peacefully amassing for us their stores of sweetness, while they lull us with their murmurs. What a beautiful image of disinterested benevolence!"

My wife declared that I was quite a poet, and the beehive was duly installed near the flower plots, that the delicate creatures might have the full benefit of the honeysuckle and mignonette. My spirits began to rise. I bought three different treatises on the rearing of bees, and also one or two new patterns of hives, and proposed to rear my bees on the most approved model. I charged all the establishment to let me know when there was any indication of an emigrating spirit, that I might be ready to receive the new swarm into my patent mansion.

Accordingly, one afternoon, when I was deep in an article that I was preparing for the "North American Review," intelligence was brought me that a swarm had risen. I was on the alert at once, and discovered, on going out, that the provoking creatures had chosen the top of a tree about thirty feet high to settle on. Now my books had carefully instructed me just how to approach the swarm and cover them with a new hive; but I had never contemplated the possibility of the swarm being, like Haman's gallows, forty cubits high. I looked despairingly upon the smooth-bark tree, which rose, like a column, full twenty feet, without branch or twig. "What is to be done?" said I, appealing to two or three neighbours. At last, at the recommendation of one of them, a ladder was raised against the tree, and, equipped with a shirt outside of my clothes, a green veil over my head, and a pair of leather gloves on my hands, I went up with a saw at my girdle to saw off the branch on which they had settled, and lower it by a rope to a neighbour, similarly equipped, who stood below with the hive.

As a result of this manoeuvre the fastidious little insects were at length fairly installed at housekeeping in my new patent hive, and, rejoicing in my success, I again sat down to my article.

That evening my wife and I took tea in our honeysuckle arbour, with our little ones and a friend or two, to whom I showed my treasures, and expatiated at large on the comforts and conveniences of the new patent hive.

But alas for the hopes of man! The little ungrateful wretches—what must they do but take advantage of my oversleeping myself, the next morning, to clear out for new quarters without so much as leaving me a P. P. C.! Such was the fact; at eight o'clock I found the new patent hive as good as ever; but the bees I have never seen from that day to this!

"The rascally little conservatives!" said I; "I believe they have never had a new idea from the days of Virgil down, and are entirely unprepared to appreciate improvements."

Meanwhile the seeds began to germinate in our garden, when we found, to our chagrin, that, between John Bull and Paddy, there had occurred sundry confusions in the several departments. Radishes had been planted broadcast, carrots and beets arranged in hills, and here and there a whole paper of seed appeared to have been planted bodily. My good old uncle, who, somewhat to my confusion, made me a call at this time, was greatly distressed and scandalized by the appearance of our garden. But by a deal of fussing, transplanting, and replanting, it was got into some shape and order. My uncle was rather troublesome, as careful old people are apt to be—annoying us by perpetual inquiries of what we gave for this and that, and running up provoking calculations on the final cost of matters; and we began to wish that his visits might be as short as would be convenient.

But when, on taking leave, he promised to send us a fine young cow of his own raising, our hearts rather smote us for our impatience.

"'Tain't any of your new breeds, nephew," said the old man, "yet I can say that she's a gentle, likely young crittur, and better worth forty dollars than many a one that's cried up for Ayrshire or Durham; and you shall be quite welcome to her."

We thanked him, as in duty bound, and thought that if he was full of old-fashioned notions, he was no less full of kindness and good will.

And now, with a new cow, with our garden beginning to thrive under the gentle showers of May, with our flower borders blooming, my wife and I began to think ourselves in Paradise. But alas! the same sun and rain that warmed our fruit and flowers brought up from the earth, like sulky gnomes, a vast array of purple-leaved weeds, that almost in a night seemed to cover the whole surface of the garden beds. Our gardeners both being gone, the weeding was expected to be done by me—one of the anticipated relaxations of my leisure hours.

"Well," said I, in reply to a gentle intimation from my wife, "when my article is finished, I'll take a day and weed all up clean."

Thus days slipped by, till at length the article was dispatched, and I proceeded to my garden. Amazement! Who could have possibly foreseen that anything earthly could grow so fast in a few days! There were no bounds, no alleys, no beds, no distinction of beet and carrot, nothing but a flourishing congregation of weeds nodding and bobbing in the morning breeze, as if to say, "We hope you are well, sir—we've got the ground, you see!" I began to explore, and to hoe, and to weed. Ah! did anybody ever try to clean a neglected carrot or beet bed, or bend his back in a hot sun over rows of weedy onions! He is the man to feel for my despair! How I weeded, and sweat, and sighed! till, when high noon came on, as the result of all my toils, only three beds were cleaned! And how disconsolate looked the good seed, thus unexpectedly delivered from its sheltering tares, and laid open to a broiling July sun! Every juvenile beet and carrot lay flat down wilted, and drooping, as if, like me, they had been weeding, instead of being weeded.

"This weeding is quite a serious matter," said I to my wife; "the fact is, I must have help about it!"

"Just what I was myself thinking," said my wife. "My flower borders are all in confusion, and my petunia mounds so completely overgrown, that nobody would dream what they were meant for!"

In short, it was agreed between us that we could not afford the expense of a full-grown man to keep our place; yet we must reinforce ourselves by the addition of a boy, and a brisk youngster from the vicinity was pitched upon as the happy addition. This youth was a fellow of decidedly quick parts, and in one forenoon made such a clearing in our garden that I was delighted. Bed after bed appeared to view, all cleared and dressed out with such celerity that I was quite ashamed of my own slowness, until, on examination, I discovered that he had, with great impartiality, pulled up both weeds and vegetables.

This hopeful beginning was followed up by a succession of proceedings which should be recorded for the instruction of all who seek for help from the race of boys. Such a loser of all tools, great and small; such an invariable leaver-open of all gates, and letter-down of bars; such a personification of all manner of anarchy and ill luck, had never before been seen on the estate. His time, while I was gone to the city, was agreeably diversified with roosting on the fence, swinging on the gates, making poplar whistles for the children, hunting eggs, and eating whatever fruit happened to be in season, in which latter accomplishment he was certainly quite distinguished. After about three weeks of this kind of joint gardening, we concluded to dismiss Master Tom from the firm, and employ a man.

"Things must be taken care of," said I, "and I cannot do it. 'Tis out of the question." And so the man was secured.

But I am making a long story, and may chance to outrun the sympathies of my readers. Time would fail me to tell of the distresses manifold that fell upon me—of cows dried up by poor milkers; of hens that wouldn't set at all, and hens that, despite all law and reason, would set on one egg; of hens that, having hatched families, straightway led them into all manner of high grass and weeds, by which means numerous young chicks caught premature colds and perished; and how, when I, with manifold toil, had driven one of these inconsiderate gadders into a coop, to teach her domestic habits, the rats came down upon her and slew every chick in one night; how my pigs were always practicing gymnastic exercises over the fence of the sty, and marauding in the garden. I wonder that Fourier never conceived the idea of having his garden land ploughed by pigs; for certainly they manifest quite a decided elective attraction for turning up the earth.

When autumn came, I went soberly to market, in the neighbouring city, and bought my potatoes and turnips like any other man; for, between all the various systems of gardening pursued, I was obliged to confess that my first horticultural effort was a decided failure. But though all my rural visions had proved illusive, there were some very substantial realities. My bill at the seed store, for seeds, roots, and tools, for example, had run up to an amount that was perfectly unaccountable; then there were various smaller items, such as horseshoeing, carriage mending—for he who lives in the country and does business in the city must keep his vehicle and appurtenances. I had always prided myself on being an exact man, and settling every account, great and small, with the going out of the old year; but this season I found myself sorely put to it. In fact, had not I received a timely lift from my good old uncle, I should have made a complete break down. The old gentleman's troublesome habit of ciphering and calculating, it seems, had led him beforehand to foresee that I was not exactly in the money-making line, nor likely to possess much surplus revenue to meet the note which I had given for my place; and, therefore, he quietly paid it himself, as I discovered, when, after much anxiety and some sleepless nights, I went to the holder to ask for an extension of credit.

"He was right, after all," said I to my wife; "'to live cheap in the country, a body must know how.'"

NATHANIEL HAWTHORNE

The Golden Touch

Once upon a time, there lived a very rich man, and a king besides, whose name was Midas; and he had a little daughter, whom nobody but myself ever heard of, and whose name I either never knew, or have entirely forgotten. So, because I love odd names for little girls, I choose to call her Marygold.

This King Midas was fonder of gold than of anything else in the world. He valued his royal crown chiefly because it was composed of that precious metal. If he loved anything better, or half so well, it was the one little maiden who played so merrily around her father's foot-stool. But the more Midas loved his daughter, the more did he desire and seek for wealth. He thought, foolish man! that the best thing he could possibly do for this dear child would be to bequeath her the immensest pile of yellow, glistening coin, that had ever been heaped together since the world was made. Thus, he gave all his thoughts and all his time to this one purpose. If ever he happened to gaze for an instant at the gold-tinted clouds of sunset, he wished that they were real gold, and that they could be squeezed safely into his strong box. When little Marygold ran to meet him, with a bunch of buttercups and dandelions, he used to say, "Poh, poh, child! If these flowers were as golden as they look, they would be worth the plucking!"

And yet, in his earlier days, before he was so entirely possessed of this insane desire for riches, King Midas had shown a great taste for flowers. He had planted a garden, in which grew the biggest and beautifullest and sweetest roses that any mortal ever saw or smelt. These roses were still growing in the garden, as large, as lovely, and as fragrant, as when Midas used to pass whole hours in gazing at them, and inhaling their perfume. But now, if he looked at them at all, it was only to calculate how much the garden would be worth if each of the innumerable rose-petals were a thin plate of gold. And though he once was fond of music (in spite of an idle story about his ears, which were said to resemble those of an ass), the only music for poor Midas, now, was the chink of one coin against another.

At length, as people always grow more and more foolish, unless they take care to grow wiser and wiser, Midas had got to be so exceedingly unreasonable, that he could scarcely bear to see or touch any object that was not gold. He made it his custom, therefore, to pass a large portion of every day in a dark and dreary apartment, under ground, at the basement of his palace. It was here that he kept his wealth. To this dismal hole— for it was little better than a dungeon—Midas betook himself, whenever he wanted to be particularly happy. Here, after carefully locking the door, he would take a bag of gold coin, or a gold cup as big as a washbowl, or a heavy golden bar, or a peck-measure of gold-dust, and bring them from the obscure corners of the room into the one bright and narrow sunbeam that fell from the dungeon-like window. He valued the sunbeam for no other reason but that his treasure would not shine without its help. And then would he reckon over the coins in the bag; toss up the bar, and catch it as it came down; sift the gold-dust through his fingers; look at the funny image of his own face, as reflected in the burnished circumference of the cup; and whisper to himself, "O Midas, rich King Midas, what a happy man art thou!" But it was laughable to see how the image of his face kept grinning at him, out of the polished surface of the cup. It seemed to be aware of his foolish behaviour, and to have a naughty inclination to make fun of him.

Midas called himself a happy man, but felt that he was not yet quite so happy as he might be. The very tip-top of enjoyment would never be reached, unless the whole world were to become his treasure-room, and be filled with yellow metal which should be all his own.

Now, I need hardly remind such wise little people as you are, that in the old, old times, when King Midas was alive, a great many things came to pass, which we should consider wonderful if they were to happen in our own day and country. And, on the other hand, a great many things take place nowadays, which seem not only wonderful to us, but at which the people of old times would have stared their eyes out. On the whole, I regard our own times as the strangest of the two; but, however that may be, I must go on with my story.

Midas was enjoying himself in his treasure-room, one day, as usual, when he perceived a shadow fall over the heaps of gold; and, looking suddenly up, what should he behold but the figure of a stranger, standing in the bright and narrow sunbeam! It was a young man, with a cheerful and ruddy face. Whether it was that the imagination of King Midas threw a yellow tinge over everything, or whatever the cause might be, he could not help fancying that the smile with which the stranger regarded him had a kind of golden radiance in it. Certainly, although his figure intercepted the sunshine, there was now a brighter gleam upon all the piled-up treasures than before. Even the remotest corners had their share of it, and were lighted up, when the stranger smiled, as with tips of flame and sparkles of fire.

As Midas knew that he had carefully turned the key in the lock, and that no mortal strength could possibly break into his treasure-room, he, of course, concluded that his visitor must be something more than mortal. It is no matter about telling you who he was. In those days, when the earth was comparatively a new affair, it was supposed to be often the resort of beings endowed with supernatural power, and who used to interest themselves in the joys and sorrows of men, women, and children, half playfully and half seriously. Midas had met such beings before now, and was not sorry to meet one of them again. The stranger's aspect, indeed, was so good-humoured and kindly, if not beneficent, that it would have been unreasonable to suspect him of intending any mischief. It was far more probable that he came to do Midas a favour. And what could that favour be, unless to multiply his heaps of treasure?

The stranger gazed about the room; and when his lustrous smile had glistened upon all the golden objects that were there, he turned again to Midas.

"You are a wealthy man, friend Midas!" he observed. "I doubt whether any other four walls, on earth, contain so much gold as you have contrived to pile up in this room."

"I have done pretty well,—pretty well," answered Midas, in a discontented tone. "But, after all, it is but a trifle, when you consider that it has taken me my whole life to get it together. If one could live a thousand years, he might have time to grow rich!"

"What!" exclaimed the stranger. "Then you are not satisfied?"

Midas shook his head.

"And pray what would satisfy you?" asked the stranger. "Merely for the curiosity of the thing, I should be glad to know."

Midas paused and meditated. He felt a presentiment that this stranger, with such a golden lustre in his good-humoured smile, had come hither with both the power and the purpose of gratifying his utmost wishes. Now, therefore, was the fortunate moment, when he had but to speak, and obtain whatever possible, or seemingly impossible, thing it might come into his head to ask. So he thought, and thought, and thought, and heaped up one golden mountain upon another, in his imagination, without being able to imagine them big enough. At last, a bright idea occurred to King Midas. It seemed really as bright as the glistening metal which he loved so much.

Raising his head, he looked the lustrous stranger in the face.

"Well, Midas," observed his visitor, "I see that you have at length hit upon something that will satisfy you. Tell me your wish."

"It is only this," replied Midas. "I am weary of collecting my treasures with so much trouble, and beholding the heap so diminutive, after I have done my best. I wish everything that I touch to be changed to gold!"

The stranger's smile grew so very broad, that it seemed to fill the room like an outburst of the sun, gleaming into a shadowy dell, where the yellow autumnal leaves—for so looked the lumps and particles of gold—lie strewn in the glow of light.

"The Golden Touch!" exclaimed he. "You certainly deserve credit, friend Midas, for striking out so brilliant a conception. But are you quite sure that this will satisfy you?"

"How could it fail?" said Midas.

"And will you never regret the possession of it?"

"What could induce me?" asked Midas. "I ask nothing else, to render me perfectly happy."

"Be it as you wish, then," replied the stranger, waving his hand in token of farewell. "To-morrow, at sunrise, you will find yourself gifted with the Golden Touch."

The figure of the stranger then became exceedingly bright, and Midas involuntarily closed his eyes. On opening them again, he beheld only one yellow sunbeam in the room, and, all around him, the glistening of the precious metal which he had spent his life in hoarding up.

Whether Midas slept as usual that night, the story does not say. Asleep or awake, however, his mind was probably in the state of a child's, to whom a beautiful new plaything has been promised in the morning. At any rate, day had hardly peeped over the hills, when King Midas was broad awake, and, stretching his arms out of bed, began to touch the objects that were within reach. He was anxious to prove whether the Golden Touch had really come, according to the stranger's promise. So he laid his finger on a chair by the bedside, and on various other things, but was grievously disappointed to perceive that they remained of exactly the same substance as before. Indeed, he felt very much afraid that he had only dreamed about the lustrous stranger, or else that the latter had been making game of him. And what a miserable affair would it be, if, after all his hopes, Midas must content himself with what little gold he could scrape together by ordinary means, instead of creating it by a touch!

All this while, it was only the grey of the morning, with but a streak of brightness along the edge of the sky, where Midas could not see it. He lay in a very disconsolate mood, regretting the downfall of his hopes, and kept growing sadder and sadder, until the earliest sunbeam shone through the window, and gilded the ceiling over his head. It seemed to Midas that this bright yellow sunbeam was reflected in rather a singular way on the white covering of the bed. Looking more closely, what was his astonishment and delight, when he found that this linen fabric had been transmuted to what seemed a woven texture of the purest and brightest gold! The Golden Touch had come to him with the first sunbeam!

Midas started up, in a kind of joyful frenzy, and ran about the room, grasping at everything that happened to be in his way. He seized one of the bed-posts, and it became immediately a fluted golden pillar. He pulled aside a window-curtain, in order to admit a clear spectacle of the wonders which he was performing; and the tassel grew heavy in his hand,—a mass of gold. He took up a book from the table. At his first touch, it assumed the appearance of such a splendidly bound and gilt-edged volume as one often meets with, nowadays; but, on running his fingers through the leaves, behold! it was a bundle of thin golden plates, in which all the wisdom of the book had grown illegible. He hurriedly put on his clothes, and was enraptured to see himself in a magnificent suit of gold cloth, which retained its flexibility and softness, although it burdened him a little with its weight. He drew out his handkerchief, which little Marygold had hemmed for him. That was likewise gold, with the dear child's neat and pretty stitches running all along the border, in gold thread!

Somehow or other, this last transformation did not quite please King Midas. He would rather that his little daughter's handiwork should have remained just the same as when she climbed his knee and put it into his hand.

But it was not worth while to vex himself about a trifle. Midas now took his spectacles from his pocket, and put them on his nose, in order that he might see more distinctly what he was about. In those days, spectacles for common people had not been invented, but were already worn by kings; else, how could Midas have had any? To his great perplexity, however, excellent as the glasses were, he discovered that he could not possibly see through them. But this was the most natural thing in the world; for, on taking them off, the transparent crystals turned out to be plates of yellow metal, and, of course, were worthless as spectacles, though valuable as gold. It struck Midas as rather inconvenient that, with all his wealth, he could never again be rich enough to own a pair of serviceable spectacles.

"It is no great matter, nevertheless," said he to himself, very philosophically. "We cannot expect any great good, without its being accompanied with some small inconvenience. The Golden Touch is worth the sacrifice of a pair of spectacles, at least, if not of one's very eyesight. My own eyes will serve for ordinary purposes, and little Marygold will soon be old enough to read to me."

Wise King Midas was so exalted by his good fortune, that the palace seemed not sufficiently spacious to contain him. He therefore went down stairs, and smiled, on observing that the balustrade of the staircase became a bar of burnished gold, as his hand passed over it, in his descent. He lifted the door-latch (it was brass only a moment ago, but golden when his fingers quitted it), and emerged into the garden. Here, as it happened, he found a great number of beautiful roses in full bloom, and others in all the stages of lovely bud and blossom. Very delicious was their fragrance in the morning breeze. Their delicate blush was one of the fairest sights in the world; so gentle, so modest, and so full of sweet tranquillity, did these roses seem to be.

But Midas knew a way to make them far more precious, according to his way of thinking, than roses had ever been before. So he took great pains in going from bush to bush, and exercised his magic touch most indefatigably; until every individual flower and bud, and even the worms at the heart of some of them, were changed to gold. By the time this good work was completed, King Midas was summoned to breakfast; and as the morning air had given him an excellent appetite, he made haste back to the palace.

What was usually a king's breakfast in the days of Midas, I really do not know, and cannot stop now to investigate. To the best of my belief, however, on this particular morning, the breakfast consisted of hot cakes, some nice little brook trout, roasted potatoes, fresh boiled eggs, and coffee, for King Midas himself, and a bowl of bread and milk for his daughter Marygold. At all events, this is a breakfast fit to set before a king; and, whether he had it or not, King Midas could not have had a better.

Little Marygold had not yet made her appearance. Her father ordered her to be called, and, seating himself at table, awaited the child's coming, in order to begin his own breakfast. To do Midas justice, he really loved his daughter, and loved her so much the more this morning, on account of the good fortune which had befallen him. It was not a great while before he heard her coming along the passageway crying bitterly. This circumstance surprised him, because Marygold was one of the cheerfullest little people whom you would see in a summer's day, and hardly shed a thimbleful of tears in a twelvemonth. When Midas heard her sobs, he determined to put little Marygold into better spirits, by an agreeable surprise; so, leaning across the table, he touched his daughter's bowl (which was a China one, with pretty figures all around it), and transmuted it to gleaming gold.

Meanwhile, Marygold slowly and disconsolately opened the door, and showed herself with her apron at her eyes, still sobbing as if her heart would break.

"How now, my little lady!" cried Midas. "Pray what is the matter with you, this bright morning?"

Marygold, without taking the apron from her eyes, held out her hand, in which was one of the roses which Midas had so recently transmuted.

"Beautiful!" exclaimed her father. "And what is there in this magnificent golden rose to make you cry?"

"Ah, dear father!" answered the child, as well as her sobs would let her; "it is not beautiful, but the ugliest flower that ever grew! As soon as I was dressed I ran into the garden to gather some roses for you; because I know you like them, and like them the better when gathered by your little daughter. But, oh dear, dear me! What do you think has happened? Such a misfortune! All the beautiful roses, that smelled so sweetly and had so many lovely blushes, are blighted and spoilt! They are grown quite yellow, as you see this one, and have no longer any fragrance! What can have been the matter with them?"

"Poh, my dear little girl,—pray don't cry about it!" said Midas, who was ashamed to confess that he himself had wrought the change which so greatly afflicted her. "Sit down and eat your bread and milk! You will find it easy enough to exchange a golden rose like that (which will last hundreds of years) for an ordinary one which would wither in a day."

"I don't care for such roses as this!" cried Marygold, tossing it contemptuously away. "It has no smell, and the hard petals prick my nose!"

The child now sat down to table, but was so occupied with her grief for the blighted roses that she did not even notice the wonderful transmutation of her China bowl. Perhaps this was all the better; for Marygold was accustomed to take pleasure in looking at the queer figures, and strange trees and houses, that were painted on the circumference of the bowl; and these ornaments were now entirely lost in the yellow hue of the metal.

Midas, meanwhile, had poured out a cup of coffee, and, as a matter of course, the coffee-pot, whatever metal it may have been when he took it up, was gold when he set it down. He thought to himself, that it was rather an extravagant style of splendour, in a king of his simple habits, to breakfast off a service of gold, and began to be puzzled with the difficulty of keeping his treasures safe. The cupboard and the kitchen would no longer be a secure place of deposit for articles so valuable as golden bowls and coffee-pots.

Amid these thoughts, he lifted a spoonful of coffee to his lips, and, sipping it, was astonished to perceive that, the instant his lips touched the liquid, it became molten gold, and, the next moment, hardened into a lump!

"Ha!" exclaimed Midas, rather aghast.

"What is the matter, father?" asked little Marygold, gazing at him, with the tears still standing in her eyes.

"Nothing, child, nothing!" said Midas. "Eat your milk, before it gets quite cold."

He took one of the nice little trouts on his plate, and, by way of experiment, touched its tail with his finger. To his horror, it was immediately transmuted from an admirably fried brook-trout into a gold-fish, though not one of those gold-fishes which people often keep in glass globes, as ornaments for the parlour. No; but it was really a metallic fish, and looked as if it had been very cunningly made by the nicest goldsmith in the world. Its little bones were now golden wires; its fins and tail were thin plates of gold; and there were the marks of the fork in it, and all the delicate, frothy appearance of a nicely fried fish, exactly imitated in metal. A very pretty piece of work, as you may suppose; only King Midas, just at that moment, would much rather have had a real trout in his dish than this elaborate and valuable imitation of one.

"I don't quite see," thought he to himself, "how I am to get any breakfast!"

He took one of the smoking-hot cakes, and had scarcely broken it, when, to his cruel mortification, though, a moment before, it had been of the whitest wheat, it assumed the yellow hue of Indian meal. To say the truth, if it had really been a hot Indian cake, Midas would have prized it a good deal more than he now did, when its solidity and increased weight made him too bitterly sensible that it was gold. Almost in despair, he helped himself to a boiled egg, which immediately underwent a change similar to those of the trout and the cake. The egg, indeed, might have been mistaken for one of those which the famous goose, in the story-book, was in the habit of laying; but King Midas was the only goose that had had anything to do with the matter.

"Well, this is a quandary!" thought he, leaning back in his chair, and looking quite enviously at little Marygold, who was now eating her bread and milk with great satisfaction. "Such a costly breakfast before me, and nothing that can be eaten!"

Hoping that, by dint of great dispatch, he might avoid what he now felt to be a considerable inconvenience, King Midas next snatched a hot potato, and attempted to cram it into his mouth, and swallow it in a hurry. But the Golden Touch was too nimble for him. He found his mouth full, not of mealy potato, but of solid metal, which so burnt his tongue that he roared aloud, and, jumping up from the table, began to dance and stamp about the room, both with pain and affright.

"Father, dear father!" cried little Marygold, who was a very affectionate child, "pray what is the matter? Have you burnt your mouth?"

"Ah, dear child," groaned Midas, dolefully, "I don't know what is to become of your poor father!"

And, truly, my dear little folks, did you ever hear of such a pitiable case in all your lives? Here was literally the richest breakfast that could be set before a king, and its very richness made it absolutely good for nothing. The poorest labourer, sitting down to his crust of bread and cup of water, was far better off than King Midas, whose delicate food was really worth its weight in gold. And what was to be done? Already, at breakfast, Midas was excessively hungry. Would he be less so by dinnertime? And how ravenous would be his appetite for supper, which must undoubtedly consist of the same sort of indigestible dishes as those now before him! How many days, think you, would he survive a continuance of this rich fare?

These reflections so troubled wise King Midas, that

he began to doubt whether, after all, riches are the one desirable thing in the world, or even the most desirable. But this was only a passing thought. So fascinated was Midas with the glitter of the yellow metal, that he would still have refused to give up the Golden Touch for so paltry a consideration as a breakfast. Just imagine what a price for one meal's victuals! It would have been the same as paying millions and millions of money (and as many millions more as would take forever to reckon up) for some fried trout, an egg, a potato, a hot cake, and a cup of coffee!

"It would be quite too dear," thought Midas.

Nevertheless, so great was his hunger, and the perplexity of his situation, that he again groaned aloud, and very grievously too. Our pretty Marygold could endure it no longer. She sat, a moment, gazing at her father, and trying, with all the might of her little wits, to find out what was the matter with him. Then, with a sweet and sorrowful impulse to comfort him, she started from her chair, and, running to Midas, threw her arms affectionately about his knees. He bent down and kissed her. He felt that his little daughter's love was worth a thousand times more than he had gained by the Golden Touch.

"My precious, precious Marygold!" cried he.

But Marygold made no answer.

Alas, what had he done? How fatal was the gift which the stranger bestowed! The moment the lips of Midas touched Marygold's forehead, a change had taken place. Her sweet, rosy face, so full of affection as it had been, assumed a glittering yellow colour, with yellow tear-drops congealing on her cheeks. Her beautiful brown ringlets took the same tint. Her soft and tender little form grew hard and inflexible within her father's encircling arms. Oh, terrible misfortune! The victim of his insatiable desire for wealth, little Marygold was a human child no longer, but a golden statue!

Yes, there she was, with the questioning look of love, grief, and pity, hardened into her face. It was the prettiest and most woeful sight that ever mortal saw. All the features and tokens of Marygold were there; even the beloved little dimple remained in her golden chin. But, the more perfect was the resemblance, the greater was the father's agony at beholding this golden image, which was all that was left him of a daughter. It had been a favourite phrase of Midas, whenever he felt particularly fond of the child, to say that she was worth her weight in gold. And now the phrase had become literally true. And now, at last, when it was too late, he felt how infinitely a warm and tender heart, that loved him, exceeded in value all the wealth that could be piled up betwixt the earth and sky!

It would be too sad a story, if I were to tell you how Midas, in the fullness of all his gratified desires, began to wring his hands and bemoan himself; and how he could neither bear to look at Marygold, nor yet to look away from her. Except when his eyes were fixed on the image, he could not possibly believe that she was changed to gold. But, stealing another glance, there was the precious little figure, with a yellow tear-drop on its yellow cheek, and a look so piteous and tender, that it seemed as if that very expression must needs soften the gold, and make it flesh again. This, however, could not be. So Midas had only to wring his hands, and to wish that he were the poorest man in the wide world, if the loss of all his wealth might bring back the faintest rose-colour to his dear child's face.

While he was in this tumult of despair, he suddenly beheld a stranger standing near the door. Midas bent down his head, without speaking; for he recognized the same figure which had appeared to him, the day before, in the treasure-room, and had bestowed on him this disastrous faculty of the Golden Touch. The stranger's countenance still wore a smile, which seemed to shed a yellow lustre all about the room, and gleamed on little Marygold's image, and on the other objects that had been transmuted by the touch of Midas.

"Well, friend Midas," said the stranger, "pray how do you succeed with the Golden Touch?"

Midas shook his head.

"I am very miserable," said he.

"Very miserable, indeed!" exclaimed the stranger. "And how happens that? Have I not faithfully kept my promise with you? Have you not everything that your heart desired?"

"Gold is not everything," answered Midas. "And I have lost all that my heart really cared for."

"Ah! So you have made a discovery, since yesterday?" observed the stranger. "Let us see, then. Which of these two things do you think is really worth the most,—the gift of the Golden Touch, or one cup of clear cold water?"

"O blessed water!" exclaimed Midas. "It will never moisten my parched throat again!"

"The Golden Touch," continued the stranger, "or a crust of bread?"

"A piece of bread," answered Midas, "is worth all the gold on earth!"

"The Golden Touch," asked the stranger, "or your own little Marygold, warm, soft, and loving as she was an hour ago?"

"Oh my child, my dear child!" cried poor Midas, wringing his hands. "I would not have given that one small dimple in her chin for the power of changing this whole big earth into a solid lump of gold!"

"You are wiser than you were, King Midas!" said the stranger, looking seriously at him. "Your own heart, I perceive, has not been entirely changed from flesh to gold. Were it so, your case would indeed be desperate. But you appear to be still capable of understanding that the commonest things, such as lie within everybody's grasp, are more valuable than the riches which so many mortals sigh and struggle after. Tell me, now, do you sincerely desire to rid yourself of this Golden Touch?"

"It is hateful to me!" replied Midas.

A fly settled on his nose, but immediately fell to the floor; for it, too, had become gold. Midas shuddered.

"Go, then," said the stranger, "and plunge into the river that glides past the bottom of your garden. Take likewise a vase of the same water, and sprinkle it over any object that you may desire to change back again from gold into its former substance. If you do this in earnestness and sincerity, it may possibly repair the mischief which your avarice has occasioned."

King Midas bowed low; and when he lifted his head, the lustrous stranger had vanished.

You will easily believe that Midas lost no time in snatching up a great earthen pitcher (but, alas me! it was no longer earthen after he touched it), and hastening to the river-side. As he scampered along, and forced his way through the shrubbery, it was positively marvellous to see how the foliage turned yellow behind him, as if the autumn had been there, and nowhere else. On reaching the river's brink, he plunged headlong in, without waiting so much as to pull off his shoes.

"Poof! poof! poof!" snorted King Midas, as his head emerged out of the water. "Well; this is really a refreshing bath, and I think it must have quite washed away the Golden Touch. And now for filling my pitcher!"

As he dipped the pitcher into the water, it gladdened his very heart to see it change from gold into the same good, honest earthen vessel which it had been before he touched it. He was conscious, also, of a change within himself. A cold, hard, and heavy weight seemed to have gone out of his bosom. No doubt, his heart had been gradually losing its human substance, and transmuting itself into insensible metal, but had now softened back again into flesh. Perceiving a violet, that grew on the bank of the river, Midas touched it with his finger, and was overjoyed to find that the delicate flower retained its purple hue, instead of undergoing a yellow blight. The curse of the Golden Touch had, therefore, really been removed from him.

King Midas hastened back to the palace; and, I suppose, the servants knew not what to make of it when they saw their royal master so carefully bringing home an earthen pitcher of water. But that water, which was to undo all the mischief that his folly had wrought, was more precious to Midas than an ocean of molten gold could have been. The first thing he did, as you need hardly be told, was to sprinkle it by handfuls over the golden figure of little Marygold.

No sooner did it fall on her than you would have laughed to see how the rosy colour came back to the dear child's cheek! and how she began to sneeze and sputter!—and how astonished she was to find herself dripping wet, and her father still throwing more water over her!

"Pray do not, dear father!" cried she. "See how you have wet my nice frock, which I put on only this morning!"

For Marygold did not know that she had been a little golden statue; nor could she remember anything that had happened since the moment when she ran with outstretched arms to comfort poor King Midas.

Her father did not think it necessary to tell his beloved child how very foolish he had been, but contented himself with showing how much wiser he had now grown. For this purpose, he led little Marygold into the garden, where he sprinkled all the remainder of the water over the rose-bushes, and with such good effect that above five thousand roses recovered their beautiful bloom. There were two circumstances, however, which, as long as he lived, used to put King Midas in mind of the Golden Touch. One was, that the sands of the river sparkled like gold; the other, that little Marygold's hair had now a golden tinge, which he had never observed in it before she had been transmuted by the effect of his kiss. This change of hue was really an improvement, and made Marygold's hair richer than in her babyhood.

When King Midas had grown quite an old man, and used to trot Marygold's children on his knee, he was fond of telling them this marvellous story, pretty much as I have now told it to you. And then would he stroke their glossy ringlets, and tell them that their hair, likewise, had a rich shade of gold, which they had inherited from their mother.

"And to tell you the truth, my precious little folks," quoth King Midas, diligently trotting the children all the while, "ever since that morning, I have hated the very sight of all other gold, save this!"

ALICE MOORE DUNBAR-NELSON

The Goodness of Saint Rocque

Manuela was tall and slender and graceful, and once you knew her the lithe form could never be mistaken. She walked with the easy spring that comes from a perfectly arched foot. To-day she swept swiftly down Marais Street, casting a quick glance here and there from under her heavy veil as if she feared she was being followed. If you had peered under the veil, you would have seen that Manuela's dark eyes were swollen and discoloured about the lids, as though they had known a sleepless, tearful night. There had been a picnic the day before, and as merry a crowd of giddy, chattering Creole girls and boys as ever you could see boarded the ramshackle dummy-train that puffed its way wheezily out wide Elysian Fields Street, around the lily-covered bayous, to Milneburg-on-the-Lake. Now, a picnic at Milneburg is a thing to be remembered for ever. One charters a rickety-looking, weather-beaten dancing-pavilion, built over the water, and after storing the children—for your true Creole never leaves the small folks at home—and the baskets and mothers down-stairs, the young folks go up-stairs and dance to the tune of the best band you ever heard. For what can equal the music of a violin, a guitar, a cornet, and a bass viol to trip the quadrille to at a picnic?

Then one can fish in the lake and go bathing under the prim bath-houses, so severely separated sexually, and go rowing on the lake in a trim boat, followed by

233

the shrill warnings of anxious mamans. And in the evening one comes home, hat crowned with cool grey Spanish moss, hands burdened with fantastic latanier baskets woven by the brown bayou boys, hand in hand with your dearest one, tired but happy.

At this particular picnic, however, there had been bitterness of spirit. Theophile was Manuela's own especial property, and Theophile had proven false. He had not danced a single waltz or quadrille with Manuela, but had deserted her for Claralie, blonde and petite. It was Claralie whom Theophile had rowed out on the lake; it was Claralie whom Theophile had gallantly led to dinner; it was Claralie's hat that he wreathed with Spanish moss, and Claralie whom he escorted home after the jolly singing ride in town on the little dummy-train.

Not that Manuela lacked partners or admirers. Dear no! she was too graceful and beautiful for that. There had been more than enough for her. But Manuela loved Theophile, you see, and no one could take his place. Still, she had tossed her head and let her silvery laughter ring out in the dance, as though she were the happiest of mortals, and had tripped home with Henri, leaning on his arm, and looking up into his eyes as though she adored him.

This morning she showed the traces of a sleepless night and an aching heart as she walked down Marais Street. Across wide St. Rocque Avenue she hastened. "Two blocks to the river and one below—" she repeated to herself breathlessly. Then she stood on the corner gazing about her, until with a final summoning of a desperate courage she dived through a small wicket gate into a garden of weed-choked flowers.

There was a hoarse, rusty little bell on the gate that gave querulous tongue as she pushed it open. The house that sat back in the yard was little and old and weather-beaten. Its one-story frame had once been painted, but that was a memory remote and traditional. A straggling morning-glory strove to conceal its time-ravaged face. The little walk of broken bits of brick was reddened carefully, and the one little step was scrupulously yellow-washed, which denoted that the occupants were cleanly as well as religious.

Manuela's timid knock was answered by a harsh "Entrez."

It was a small sombre room within, with a bare yellow-washed floor and ragged curtains at the little window. In a corner was a diminutive altar draped with threadbare lace. The red glow of the taper lighted a cheap print of St. Joseph and a brazen crucifix. The human element in the room was furnished by a little, wizened yellow woman, who, black-robed, turbaned, and stern, sat before an uncertain table whereon were greasy cards.

Manuela paused, her eyes blinking at the semi-obscurity within. The Wizened One called in croaking tones:

"An' fo' w'y you come here? Assiez-la, ma'amzelle."

Timidly Manuela sat at the table facing the owner of the voice.

"I want," she began faintly; but the Mistress of the Cards understood: she had had much experience. The cards were shuffled in her long grimy talons and stacked before Manuela.

"Now you cut dem in t'ree part, so—un, deux, trois, bien! You mek' you' weesh wid all you' heart, bien! Yaas, I see, I see!"

Breathlessly did Manuela learn that her lover was

true, but "dat light gal, yaas, she mek' nouvena in St. Rocque fo' hees love."

"I give you one lil' charm, yaas," said the Wizened One when the seance was over, and Manuela, all white and nervous, leaned back in the rickety chair. "I give you one lil' charm fo' to ween him back, yaas. You wear h'it 'roun' you' wais', an' he come back. Den you mek prayer at St. Rocque an' burn can'le. Den you come back an' tell me, yaas. Cinquante sous, ma'amzelle. Merci. Good luck go wid you."

Readjusting her veil, Manuela passed out the little wicket gate, treading on air. Again the sun shone, and the breath of the swamps came as healthful sea-breeze unto her nostrils. She fairly flew in the direction of St. Rocque.

There were quite a number of persons entering the white gates of the cemetery, for this was Friday, when all those who wish good luck pray to the saint, and wash their steps promptly at twelve o'clock with a wondrous mixture to guard the house. Manuela bought a candle from the keeper of the little lodge at the entrance, and pausing one instant by the great sun-dial to see if the heavens and the hour were propitious, glided into the tiny chapel, dim and stifling with heavy air from myriad wish-candles blazing on the wide table before the altar-rail. She said her prayer and lighting her candle placed it with the others.

Mon Dieu! how brightly the sun seemed to shine now, she thought, pausing at the door on her way out. Her small finger-tips, still bedewed with holy water, rested caressingly on a gamin's head. The ivy which enfolds the quaint chapel never seemed so green; the shrines which serve as the Way of the Cross never seemed so artistic; the baby graves, even, seemed cheerful.

Theophile called Sunday. Manuela's heart leaped. He had been spending his Sundays with Claralie. His stay was short and he was plainly bored. But Manuela knelt to thank the good St. Rocque that night, and fondled the charm about her slim waist. There came a box of bonbons during the week, with a decorative card all roses and fringe, from Theophile; but being a Creole, and therefore superstitiously careful, and having been reared by a wise and experienced maman to mistrust the gifts of a recreant lover, Manuela quietly thrust bonbons, box, and card into the kitchen fire, and the Friday following placed the second candle of her nouvena in St. Rocque.

Those of Manuela's friends who had watched with indignation Theophile gallantly leading Claralie home from High Mass on Sundays, gasped with astonishment when the next Sunday, with his usual bow, the young man offered Manuela his arm as the worshippers filed out in step to the organ's march. Claralie tossed her head as she crossed herself with holy water, and the pink in her cheeks was brighter than usual.

Manuela smiled a bright good-morning when she met Claralie in St. Rocque the next Friday. The little blonde blushed furiously, and Manuela rushed post-haste to the Wizened One to confer upon this new issue.

"H'it ees good," said the dame, shaking her turbaned head. "She ees 'fraid, she will work, mais you' charm, h'it weel beat her."

And Manuela departed with radiant eyes.

Theophile was not at Mass Sunday morning, and murderous glances flashed from Claralie to Manuela before the tinkling of the Host-Bell. Nor did Theophile call at either house. Two hearts beat furiously at the sound of every passing footstep, and two minds wondered if the other were enjoying the beloved one's smiles. Two pair of eyes, however, blue and black, smiled on others, and their owners laughed and seemed none the less happy. For your Creole girls are proud, and would die rather than let the world see their sorrows.

Monday evening Theophile, the missing, showed his rather sheepish countenance in Manuela's parlour, and explained that he, with some chosen spirits, had gone for a trip—"over the Lake."

"I did not ask you where you were yesterday," replied the girl, saucily.

Theophile shrugged his shoulders and changed the conversation.

The next week there was a birthday fete in honour of Louise, Theophile's young sister. Everyone was bidden, and no one thought of refusing, for Louise was young, and this would be her first party. So, though the night was hot, the dancing went on as merrily as light young feet could make it go. Claralie fluffed her dainty white skirts, and cast mischievous sparkles in the direction of Theophile, who with the maman and Louise was bravely trying not to look self-conscious. Manuela, tall and calm and proud-looking, in a cool, pale yellow gown was apparently enjoying herself without paying the slightest attention to her young host.

"Have I the pleasure of this dance?" he asked her finally, in a lull of the music.

She bowed assent, and as if moved by a common impulse they strolled out of the dancing-room into the cool, quaint garden, where jessamines gave out an overpowering perfume, and a caged mocking-bird complained melodiously to the full moon in the sky.

It must have been an engrossing tete-a-tete, for the call to supper had sounded twice leading on the arm of papa. Claralie tripped by with Leon. Of course, nothing remained for Theophile and Manuela to do but to bring up the rear, for which they received much good-natured chaffing.

But when the party reached the dining-room, Theophile proudly led his partner to the head of the table, at the right hand of maman, and smiled benignly about at the delighted assemblage. Now you know, when a Creole young man places a girl at his mother's right hand at his own table, there is but one conclusion to be deduced therefrom.

If you had asked Manuela, after the wedding was over, how it happened, she would have said nothing, but looked wise.

If you had asked Claralie, she would have laughed and said she always preferred Leon.

If you had asked Theophile, he would have wondered that you thought he had ever meant more than to tease Manuela.

If you had asked the Wizened One, she would have offered you a charm.

But St. Rocque knows, for he is a good saint, and if you believe in him and are true and good, and make your nouvenas with a clean heart, he will grant your wish.

MARK TWAIN

Jim Baker's Blue Jay Yarn

Animals talk to each other, of course. There can be no question about that; but I suppose there are very few people who can understand them. I never knew but one man who could. I knew he could, however, because he told me so himself. He was a middle-aged, simple-hearted miner who had lived in a lonely corner of California, among the woods and mountains, a good many years, and had studied the ways of his only neighbours, the beasts and the birds, until he believed he could accurately translate any remark which they made. This was Jim Baker. According to Jim Baker, some animals have only a limited education, and some use only simple words, and scarcely ever a comparison or a flowery figure; whereas, certain other animals have a large vocabulary, a fine command of language and a ready and fluent delivery; consequently these latter talk a great deal; they like it; they are so conscious of their talent, and they enjoy "showing off." Baker said, that after long and careful observation, he had come to the conclusion that the blue jays were the best talkers he had found among birds and beasts. Said he:

"There's more *to* a blue jay than any other creature. He has got more moods, and more different kinds of feelings than other creatures; and, mind you, whatever a blue jay feels, he can put into language. And no mere commonplace language, either, but rattling, out-and-out book-talk—and bristling with metaphor, too—just bristling! And as for command of language—why *you* never see a blue jay get stuck for a word. No man ever did. They just boil out of him! And another thing: I've noticed a good deal, and there's no bird, or cow, or anything that uses as good grammar as a blue jay. You may say a cat uses good grammar. Well, a cat does—but you let a cat get excited once; you let a cat get to pulling fur with another cat on a shed, nights, and you'll hear grammar that will give you the lockjaw. Ignorant people think it's the *noise* which fighting cats make that is so aggravating, but it ain't so; it's the sickening grammar they use. Now I've never heard a jay use bad grammar but very seldom; and when they do, they are as ashamed as a human; they shut right down and leave.

"You may call a jay a bird. Well, so he is, in a measure—but he's got feathers on him, and don't belong to no church, perhaps; but otherwise he is just as much human as you be. And I'll tell you for why. A jay's gifts, and instincts, and feelings, and interests, cover the whole ground. A jay hasn't got any more principle than a Congressman. A jay will lie, a jay will steal, a jay will deceive, a jay will betray; and four times out of five, a jay will go back on his solemnest promise. The sacredness of an obligation is such a thing which you can't cram into no blue jay's head. Now, on top of all this, there's another thing; a jay can out-swear any gentleman in the mines. You think a cat can swear. Well, a cat can; but you give a blue jay a subject that calls for his reserve-powers, and where is your cat? Don't talk to *me*—I know too much about this thing; in the one little particular of scolding—just good, clean, out-and-out scolding—a blue jay can lay over anything, human or divine. Yes, sir, a jay is everything that a man is. A jay can cry, a jay can laugh, a jay can feel shame, a jay can reason and plan and discuss, a jay likes gossip and scandal, a jay has got a sense of humour, a jay knows when he is an ass just as well as you do—maybe better. If a jay ain't human, he better take in his sign, that's all. Now I'm going to tell you a perfectly true fact about some blue jays.

"When I first begun to understand jay language correctly, there was a little incident happened here. Seven years ago, the last man in this region but me moved away. There stands his house—been empty ever since; a log house, with a plank roof—just one big room, and no more; no ceiling—nothing between the rafters and the floor. Well, one Sunday morning I was sitting out here in front of my cabin, with my cat, taking the sun, and looking at the blue hills, and listening to the leaves rustling so lonely in the trees, and thinking of the home away yonder in the states, that I hadn't heard from in thirteen years, when a blue jay lit on that house, with an acorn in his mouth, and says, 'Hello, I reckon I've struck something.' When he spoke, the acorn dropped out of his mouth and rolled down the roof, of course, but he didn't care; his mind was all on the thing he had struck. It was a knot-hole in the roof. He cocked his head to one side, shut one eye and put the other one to the hole, like a possum looking down a jug; then he glanced up with his bright eyes, gave a wink or two with his wings—which signifies gratification, you understand—and says, 'It looks like a hole, it's located like a hole—blamed if I don't believe it *is* a hole!'

"Then he cocked his head down and took another look; he glances up perfectly joyful, this time; winks his wings and his tail both, and says, 'Oh, no, this ain't no fat thing, I reckon! If I ain't in luck!—Why it's a perfectly elegant hole!' So he flew down and got that acorn, and fetched it up and dropped it in, and was just tilting his head back, with the heavenliest smile on his face, when all of a sudden he was paralyzed into a listening attitude and that smile faded gradually out of his countenance like breath off'n a razor, and the queerest look of surprise took its place. Then he says, 'Why, I didn't hear it fall!' He cocked his eye at the hole again, and took a long look; raised up and shook his head; stepped around to the other side of the hole and took another look from that side; shook his head again. He studied a while, then he just went into the *details*—walked round and round the hole and spied into it from every point of the compass. No use. Now he took a thinking attitude on the comb of the roof and scratched the back of his head with his right foot a minute, and finally says, 'Well, it's too many for *me*, that's certain; must be a mighty long hole; however, I ain't got no time to fool around here, I got to "tend to business"; I reckon it's all right—chance it, anyway.'

"So he flew off and fetched another acorn and dropped it in, and tried to flirt his eye to the hole quick enough to see what become of it, but he was too late. He held his eye there as much as a minute; then he raised up and sighed, and says, 'Confound it, I don't seem to understand this thing, no way; however, I'll tackle her again.' He fetched another acorn, and done his level best to see what become of it, but he couldn't. He says, 'Well, I never struck no such a hole as this before; I'm of the opinion it's a totally new kind of a hole.' Then he begun to get mad. He held in for a spell, walking up and down the comb of the roof and shaking his head and muttering to himself; but his feelings got the upper hand of him, presently, and he broke loose and cussed himself black in the face. I never see a bird take on so about a little thing. When he got through he walks to the hole and looks in again for half a minute; then he says, 'Well, you're a long hole, and a deep hole, and a mighty singular hole altogether—but I've started in to fill you, and I'm damned if I *don't* fill you, if it takes a hundred years!'

"And with that, away he went. You never see a bird work so since you was born. He laid into his work, and the way he hove acorns into that hole for about two hours and a half was one of the most exciting and astonishing spectacles I ever struck. He never stopped to take a look anymore—he just hove 'em in and went for more. Well, at last he could hardly flop his wings, he was so tuckered out. He comes a-dropping down, once more, sweating like an ice-pitcher, dropped his acorn in and says, '*Now* I guess I've got the bulge on you by this time!' So he bent down for a look. If you'll believe me, when his head come up again he was just pale with rage. He says, 'I've shovelled acorns enough in there to keep the family thirty years, and if I can see a sign of one of 'em I wish I may land in a museum with a belly full of sawdust in two minutes!'

"He just had strength enough to crawl up on to the comb and lean his back agin the chimbly, and then he collected his impressions and begun to free his mind. I see in a second that what I had mistook for profanity in the mines was only just the rudiments, as you may say.

"Another jay was going by, and heard him doing his devotions, and stops to inquire what was up. The sufferer told him the whole circumstance, and says, 'Now yonder's the hole, and if you don't believe me, go and look for yourself.' So this fellow went and looked, and comes back and says, 'How many did you say you put in there?' 'Not any less than two tons,' says the sufferer. The other jay went and looked again. He couldn't seem to make it out, so he raised a yell, and three more jays come. They all examined the hole, they all made the sufferer tell it over again, then they all discussed it, and got off as many leather-headed opinions about it as an average crowd of humans could have done.

"They called in more jays; then more and more, till pretty soon this whole region 'peared to have a blue flush about it. There must have been five thousand of them; and such another jawing and disputing and ripping and cussing, you never heard. Every jay in the whole lot put his eye to the hole and delivered a more chuckle-headed opinion about the mystery than the jay that went there before him. They examined the house all over, too. The door was standing half open, and at last one old jay happened to go and light on it and look in. Of course, that knocked the mystery galley-west in a second. There lay the acorns, scattered all over the floor.. He flopped his wings and raised a whoop. 'Come here!' he says, 'Come here, everybody; hang'd if this fool hasn't been trying to fill up a house with acorns!' They all came a-swooping down like a blue cloud, and as each fellow lit on the door and took a glance, the whole absurdity of the contract that that first jay had tackled hit him home and he fell over backward suffocating with laughter, and the next jay took his place and done the same.

"Well, sir, they roosted around here on the housetop and the trees for an hour, and guffawed over that thing like human beings. It ain't any use to tell me a blue jay hasn't got a sense of humour, because I know better. And memory, too. They brought jays here from all over the United States to look down that hole, every summer for three years. Other birds, too. And they could all see the point except an owl that come from

Nova Scotia to visit the Yosemite, and he took this thing in on his way back. He said he couldn't see anything funny in it. But then he was a good deal disappointed about Yosemite, too."

L. M. Montgomery

The Garden of Spices

Jims tried the door of the blue room. Yes, it was locked.
He had hoped Aunt Augusta *might* have forgotten to
lock it; but when did Aunt Augusta forget anything?
Except, perhaps, that little boys were not born grown-
ups—and *that* was something she never remembered.
To be sure, she was only a half-aunt. Whole aunts probably had more convenient memories.

Jims turned and stood with his back against the door.
It was better that way; he could not imagine things
behind him then. And the blue room was so big and
dim that a dreadful number of things could be imag-
ined in it. All the windows were shuttered but one, and
that one was so darkened by a big pine tree branching
right across it that it did not let in much light.

Jims looked very small and lost and lonely as he
shrank back against the door—so small and lonely that
one might have thought that even the sternest of half-
aunts should have thought twice before shutting him up
in that room and telling him he must stay there the
whole afternoon instead of going out for a promised
ride. Jims hated being shut up alone—especially in the
blue room. Its bigness and dimness and silence filled his
sensitive little soul with vague horror. Sometimes he
became almost sick with fear in it. To do Aunt Augusta
justice, she never suspected this. If she had she would
not have decreed this particular punishment, because
she knew Jims was delicate and must not be subjected to

any great physical or mental strain. That was why she shut him up instead of whipping him. But how was she to know it? Aunt Augusta was one of those people who never know anything unless it is told them in plain language and then hammered into their heads. There was no one to tell her but Jims, and Jims would have died the death before he would have told Aunt Augusta, with her cold, spectacled eyes and thin, smileless mouth, that he was desperately frightened when he was shut in the blue room. So he was always shut in it for punishment; and the punishments came very often, for Jims was always doing things that Aunt Augusta considered naughty. At first, this time, Jims did not feel quite so frightened as usual because he was very angry. As he put it, he was very mad at Aunt Augusta. He hadn't *meant* to spill his pudding over the floor and the tablecloth and his clothes; and how such a little bit of pudding—Aunt Augusta was mean with desserts—could ever have spread itself over so much territory Jims could not understand. But he had made a terrible mess and Aunt Augusta had been very angry and had said he must be cured of such carelessness. She said he must spend the afternoon in the blue room instead of going for a ride with Mrs. Loring in her new car.

Jims was bitterly disappointed. If Uncle Walter had been home Jims would have appealed to him—for when Uncle Walter could be really wakened up to a realization of his small nephew's presence in his home, he was very kind and indulgent. But it was so hard to waken him up that Jims seldom attempted it. He liked Uncle Walter, but as far as being acquainted with him went he might as well have been the inhabitant of a star in the Milky Way. Jims was just a lonely, solitary little creature, and sometimes he felt so friendless that his eyes smarted, and several sobs had to be swallowed.

There were no sobs just now, though—Jims was still too angry. It wasn't fair. It was so seldom he got a car ride. Uncle Walter was always too busy, attending to sick children all over the town, to take him. It was only once in a blue moon Mrs. Loring asked him to go out with her. But she always ended up with ice cream or a movie, and to-day Jims had had strong hopes that both were on the programme.

"I hate Aunt Augusta," he said aloud; and then the sound of his voice in that huge, still room scared him so that he only thought the rest. "I won't have any fun—and she won't feed my gobbler, either."

Jims had shrieked "Feed my gobbler," to the old servant as he had been hauled upstairs. But he didn't think Nancy Jane had heard him, and nobody, not even Jims, could imagine Aunt Augusta feeding the gobbler. It was always a wonder to him that she ate, herself. It seemed really too human a thing for her to do.

"I wish I had spilled that pudding *on purpose*," Jims said vindictively, and with the saying his anger evaporated—Jims never could stay angry long—and left him merely a scared little fellow, with velvety, nut-brown eyes full of fear that should have no place in a child's eyes. He looked so small and helpless as he crouched against the door that one might have wondered if even Aunt Augusta would not have relented had she seen him.

How that window at the far end of the room rattled! It sounded terribly as if somebody—or *something*—were trying to get in. Jims looked desperately at the unshuttered window. He must get to it; once there, he could curl up in the window seat, his back to the wall, and forget the shadows by looking out into the sunshine and loveliness of the garden over the wall. Jims would have likely have been found dead of fright in that blue room some time had it not been for the garden over the wall.

But to get to the window Jims must cross the room and pass by the bed. Jims held that bed in special dread. It was the oldest fashioned thing in the old-fashioned, old-furnitured house. It was high and rigid, and hung with gloomy blue curtains. *Anything* might jump out of such a bed.

Jims gave a gasp and ran madly across the room. He reached the window and flung himself upon the seat. With a sigh of relief he curled down in the corner. Outside, over the high brick wall, was a world where his imagination could roam, though his slender little body was pent a prisoner in the blue room.

Jims had loved that garden from his first sight of it. He called it the Garden of Spices and wove all sorts of yarns in fancy—yarns gay and tragic—about it. He had only known it for a few weeks. Before that, they had lived in a much smaller house away at the other side of the town. Then Uncle Walter's uncle—who had brought him up just as he was bringing up Jims—had died, and they had all come to live in Uncle Walter's old home. Somehow, Jims had an idea that Uncle Walter wasn't very glad to come back there. But he had to, according to great-uncle's will. Jims himself didn't mind much. He liked the smaller rooms in their former home better, but the Garden of Spices made up for all.

It was such a beautiful spot. Just inside the wall was a row of aspen poplars that always talked in silvery whispers and shook their dainty, heart-shaped leaves at him. Beyond them, under scattered pines, was a rockery where ferns and wild things grew. It was almost as good as a bit of woods—and Jims loved the woods, though he scarcely ever saw them. Then, past the pines, were roses just breaking into June bloom—roses in such profusion as Jims hadn't known existed, with dear little paths twisting about among the bushes. It seemed to be a garden where no frost could blight or rough wind blow. When rain fell it must fall very gently. Past the roses one saw a green lawn, sprinkled over now with the white ghosts of dandelions, and dotted with ornamental trees. The trees grew so thickly that they almost hid the house to which the garden pertained. It was a large one of grey-black stone, with stacks of huge chimneys. Jims had no idea who lived there. He had asked Aunt Augusta and Aunt Augusta had frowned and told him it did not matter who lived there and that he must never, on any account, mention the next house or its occupant to Uncle Walter. Jims would never have thought of mentioning them to Uncle Walter. But the prohibition filled him with an unholy and unsubduable curiosity. He was devoured by the desire to find out who the folks in that tabooed house were.

And he longed to have the freedom of that garden. Jims loved gardens. There had been a garden at the little house but there was none here—nothing but an old lawn that had been fine once but was now badly run to seed. Jims had heard Uncle Walter say that he was going to have it attended to but nothing had been done yet. And meanwhile here was a beautiful garden over the wall which looked as if it should be full of children. But no children were ever in it—or anybody else apparently. And so, in spite of its beauty, it had a lonely look that hurt Jims. He *wanted* his Garden of Spices to be full of laughter. He pictured himself running in it with imaginary playmates—and there was a mother in it—or a big sister—or, at the least, a whole aunt who would let you hug her and would never dream of shutting you up in chilly, shadowy, horrible blue rooms.

"It seems to me," said Jims, flattening his nose against the pane, "that I must get into that garden or bust."

Aunt Augusta would have said icily, "We do not use such expressions, James," but Aunt Augusta was not there to hear.

"I'm afraid the Very Handsome Cat isn't coming to-day," sighed Jims. Then he brightened up; the Very Handsome Cat was coming across the lawn. He was the only living thing, barring birds and butterflies, that Jims ever saw in the garden. Jims worshipped that cat. He was jet black, with white paws and dickey, and he had as much dignity as ten cats. Jims' fingers tingled to stroke him. Jims had never been allowed to have even a kitten because Aunt Augusta had a horror of cats. And you cannot stroke gobblers!

The Very Handsome Cat came through the rose garden paths on his beautiful paws, ambled daintily around the rockery, and sat down in a shady spot under a pine tree, right where Jims could see him, through a gap in the little poplars. He looked straight up at Jims and winked. At least, Jims always believed and declared he did. And that wink said, or seemed to say, plainly:

"Be a sport. Come down here and play with me. A fig for your Aunt Augusta!"

A wild, daring, absurd idea flashed into Jims' brain. Could he? He could! He would! He knew it would be easy. He had thought it all out many times, although until now he had never dreamed of really doing it. To unhook the window and swing it open, to step out on the pine bough and from it to another that hung over the wall and dropped nearly to the ground, to spring from it to the velvet sward under the poplars—why, it was all the work of a minute. With a careful, repressed whoop Jims ran towards the Very Handsome Cat.

The cat rose and retreated in deliberate haste; Jims ran after him. The cat dodged through the rose paths and eluded Jims' eager hands, just keeping tantalizingly out of reach. Jims had forgotten everything except that he must catch the cat. He was full of a fearful joy, with an elfin delight running through it. He had escaped from the blue room and its ghosts; he was in his Garden of Spices; he had got the better of mean old Aunt Augusta. But he *must* catch the cat.

The cat ran over the lawn and Jims pursued it through the green gloom of the thickly clustering trees. Beyond them came a pool of sunshine in which the old stone house basked like a huge grey cat itself. More garden was before it and beyond it, wonderful with blossom. Under a huge spreading beech tree in the centre of it was a little tea table; sitting by the table reading was a lady in a black dress.

The cat, having lured Jims to where he wanted him, sat down and began to lick his paws. He was quite willing to be caught now; but Jims had no longer any idea of catching him. He stood very still, looking at the lady. She did not see him then and Jims could only see her profile, which he thought very beautiful. She had wonderful ropes of blue-black hair wound around her head. She looked so sweet that Jims' heart beat. Then she lifted her head and turned her face and saw him. Jims felt something of a shock. She was not pretty after all. One side of her face was marked by a dreadful red scar.

It quite spoilt her good looks, which Jims thought a great pity; but nothing could spoil the sweetness of her face or the loveliness of her peculiar soft, grey-blue eyes. Jims couldn't remember his mother and had no idea what she looked like, but the thought came into his head that he would have liked her to have eyes like that. After the first moment Jims did not mind the scar at all.

But perhaps that first moment had revealed itself in his face, for a look of pain came into the lady's eyes and, almost involuntarily it seemed, she put her hand up to hide the scar. Then she pulled it away again and sat looking at Jims half defiantly, half piteously. Jims thought she must be angry because he had chased her cat.

"I beg your pardon," he said gravely, "I didn't mean to hurt your cat. I just wanted to play with him. He is *such* a very handsome cat."

"But where did you come from?" said the lady. "It is so long since I saw a child in this garden," she added, as if to herself. Her voice was as sweet as her face. Jims thought he was mistaken in thinking her angry and plucked up heart of grace. Shyness was no fault of Jims.

"I came from the house over the wall," he said. "My name is James Brander Churchill. Aunt Augusta shut me up in the blue room because I spilled my pudding at dinner. I hate to be shut up. And I was to have had a ride this afternoon—and ice cream—and *maybe* a movie. So I was mad. And when your Very Handsome Cat came and looked at me I just got out and climbed down."

He looked straight at her and smiled. Jims had a very dear little smile. It seemed a pity there was no mother alive to revel in it. The lady smiled back.

"I think you did right," she said.

"*You* wouldn't shut a little boy up if you had one, would you?" said Jims.

"No—no, dear heart, I wouldn't," said the lady. She said it as if something hurt her horribly. She smiled again gallantly.

"Will you come here and sit down?" she added, pulling a chair out from the table.

"Thank you. I'd rather sit here," said Jims, plumping down on the grass at her feet. "Then maybe your cat will come to me."

The cat came over promptly and rubbed his head against Jims' knee. Jims stroked him delightedly; how lovely his soft fur felt and his round velvety head.

"I like cats," explained Jims, "and I have nothing but a gobbler. This is such a Very Handsome Cat. What is his name, please?"

"Black Prince. He loves me," said the lady. "He always comes to my bed in the morning and wakes me by patting my face with his paw. *He* doesn't mind my being ugly."

She spoke with a bitterness Jims couldn't understand.

"But you are not ugly," he said.

"Oh, I *am* ugly—I *am* ugly," she cried. "Just look at me—right at me. Doesn't it hurt you to look at me?"

Jims looked at her gravely and dispassionately.

"No, it doesn't," he said. "Not a bit," he added, after some further exploration of his consciousness.

Suddenly the lady laughed beautifully. A faint rosy flush came into her unscarred cheek.

"James, I believe you mean it."

"Of course I mean it. And, if you don't mind, please call me Jims. Nobody calls me James but Aunt Augusta. She isn't my whole aunt. She is just Uncle Walter's half-sister. *He* is my whole uncle."

"What does he call you?" asked the lady. She looked away as she asked it.

"Oh, Jims, when he thinks about me. He doesn't often think about me. He has too many sick children to think about. Sick children are all Uncle Walter cares about. He's the greatest children's doctor in the Dominion, Mr. Burroughs says. But he is a woman-hater."

"How do you know that?"

"Oh, I heard Mr. Burroughs say it. Mr. Burroughs is my tutor, you know. I study with him from nine till one. I'm not allowed to go to the public school. I'd like to, but Uncle Walter thinks I'm not strong enough yet. I'm going next year, though, when I'm ten. I have holidays now. Mr. Burroughs always goes away the first of June."

"How came he to tell you your uncle was a woman-hater?" persisted the lady.

"Oh, he didn't tell me. He was talking to a friend of his. He thought I was reading my book. So I was—but I heard it all. It was more interesting than my book. Uncle Walter was engaged to a lady, long, long ago, when he was a young man. She was devilishly pretty."

"Oh, Jims!"

"Mr. Burroughs said so. I'm only quoting," said Jims easily. "And Uncle Walter just worshipped her. And all at once she just jilted him without a word of explanation, Mr. Burroughs said. So that is why he hates women. It isn't any wonder, is it?"

"I suppose not," said the lady with a sigh. "Jims, are you hungry?"

"Yes, I am. You see, the pudding was spilled. But how did you know?"

"Oh, boys always used to be hungry when I knew them long ago. I thought they hadn't changed. I shall tell Martha to bring out something to eat and we'll have it here under this tree. You sit here—I'll sit there. Jims, it's so long since I talked to a little boy that I'm not sure that I know how."

"You know how, all right," Jims assured her. "But what am I to call you, please?"

"My name is Miss Garland," said the lady a little hesitatingly. But she saw the name meant nothing to Jims. "I would like you to call me Miss Avery. Avery is my first name and I never hear it nowadays. Now for a jamboree! I can't offer you a movie—and I'm afraid there isn't any ice cream either. I could have had some if I'd known you were coming. But I think Martha will be able to find something good."

A very old woman, who looked at Jims with great amazement, came out to set the table. Jims thought she must be as old as Methuselah. But he did not mind her. He ran races with Black Prince while tea was being prepared, and rolled the delighted cat over and over in the grass. And he discovered a fragrant herb-garden in a far corner and was delighted. Now it was truly a garden of spices.

"Oh, it is so beautiful here," he told Miss Avery, who sat and looked at his revels with a hungry expression in her lovely eyes. "I wish I could come often."

"Why can't you?" said Miss Avery.

The two looked at each other with sly intelligence.

"I could come whenever Aunt Augusta shuts me up in the blue room," said Jims.

"Yes," said Miss Avery. Then she laughed and held out her arms. Jims flew into them. He put his arms about her neck and kissed her scarred face.

"Oh, I wish *you* were my aunt," he said.

Miss Avery suddenly pushed him away. Jims was

horribly afraid he had offended her. But she took his hand.

"We'll just be chums, Jims," she said. "That's really better than being relations, after all. Come and have tea."

Over that glorious tea-table they became life-long friends. They had always known each other and always would. The Black Prince sat between them and was fed tit-bits. There was such a lot of good things on the table and nobody to say "You have had enough, James." James ate until *he* thought he had enough. Aunt Augusta would have thought he was doomed, could she have seen him.

"I suppose I must go back," said Jims with a sigh. "It will be our supper time in half an hour and Aunt Augusta will come to take me out."

"But you'll come again?"

"Yes, the first time she shuts me up. And if she doesn't shut me up pretty soon I'll be so bad she'll have to shut me up."

"I'll always set a place for you at the tea-table after this, Jims. And when you're not here I'll pretend you are. And when you can't come here write me a letter and bring it when you do come."

"Good-bye," said Jims. He took her hand and kissed it. He had read of a young knight doing that and had always thought he would like to try it if he ever got a chance. But who could dream of kissing Aunt Augusta's hands?

"You dear, funny thing," said Miss Avery. "Have you thought of how you are to get back? Can you reach that pine bough from the ground?"

"Maybe I can jump," said Jims dubiously.

"I'm afraid not. I'll give you a stool and you can

stand on it. Just leave it there for future use. Good-bye, Jims. Jims, two hours ago I didn't know there was such a person in the world as you—and now I love you—I love you."

Jims' heart filled with a great warm gush of gladness. He had always wanted to be loved. And no living creature, he felt sure, loved him, except his gobbler—and a gobbler's love is not very satisfying, though it is better than nothing. He was blissfully happy as he carried his stool across the lawn. He climbed his pine and went in at the window and curled up on the seat in a maze of delight. The blue room was more shadowy than ever but that did not matter. Over in the Garden of Spices was friendship and laughter and romance galore. The whole world was transformed for Jims.

From that time Jims lived a shamelessly double life. Whenever he was shut in the blue room he escaped to the Garden of Spices—and he was shut in very often, for, Mr. Burroughs being away, he got into a good deal of what Aunt Augusta called mischief. Besides, it is a sad truth that Jims didn't try very hard to be good now. He thought it paid better to be bad and be shut up. To be sure there was always a fly in the ointment. He was haunted by a vague fear that Aunt Augusta might relent and come to the blue room before supper time to let him out.

"And *then* the fat would be in the fire," said Jims.

But he had a glorious summer and throve so well on his new diet of love and companionship that one day Uncle Walter, with fewer sick children to think about than usual, looked at him curiously and said:

"Augusta, that boy seems to be growing much stronger. He has a good colour and his eyes are getting to look more like a boy's eyes should. We'll make a man of you yet, Jims."

"He may be getting stronger but he's getting naughtier, too," said Aunt Augusta, grimly. "I am sorry to say, Walter, that he behaves very badly."

"We were all young once," said Uncle Walter indulgently.

"Were *you*?" asked Jims in blank amazement.

Uncle Walter laughed.

"Do you think me an antediluvian, Jims?"

"I don't know what *that* is. But your hair is grey and your eyes are tired," said Jims uncompromisingly.

Uncle Walter laughed again, tossed Jims a quarter, and went out.

"Your uncle is only forty-five and in his prime," said Aunt Augusta dourly.

Jims deliberately ran across the room to the window and, under pretence of looking out, knocked down a flower pot. So he was exiled to the blue room and got into his beloved Garden of Spices where Miss Avery's beautiful eyes looked love into his and the Black Prince was a jolly playmate and old Martha petted and spoiled him to her heart's content.

Jims never asked questions but he was a wide-awake chap, and, taking one thing with another, he found out a good deal about the occupants of the old stone house. Miss Avery never went anywhere and no one ever went there. She lived all alone with two old servants, man and maid. Except these two and Jims nobody had ever seen her for twenty years. Jims didn't know why, but he thought it must be because of the scar on her face.

He never referred to it, but one day Miss Avery told him what caused it.

"I dropped a lamp and my dress caught fire and

burned my face, Jims. It made me hideous. I was beautiful before that—very beautiful. Everybody said so. Come in and I will show you my picture."

She took him into her big parlour and showed him the picture hanging on the wall between the two high windows. It was of a young girl in white. She certainly was very lovely, with her rose-leaf skin and laughing eyes. Jims looked at the pictured face gravely, with his hands in his pockets and his head on one side. Then he looked at Miss Avery.

"You were prettier then—yes," he said, judicially, "but I like your face ever so much better now."

"Oh, Jims, you can't," she protested.

"Yes, I do," persisted Jims. "You look kinder and—nicer now."

It was the nearest Jims could get to expressing what he felt as he looked at the picture. The young girl was beautiful, but her face was a little hard. There was pride and vanity and something of the insolence of great beauty in it. There was nothing of that in Miss Avery's face now—nothing but sweetness and tenderness, and a motherly yearning to which every fibre of Jims' small being responded. How they loved each other, those two! And how they understood each other! To *love* is easy, and therefore common; but to *understand*—how rare that is! And oh! such good times as they had! They made taffy. Jims had always longed to make taffy, but Aunt Augusta's immaculate kitchen and saucepans might not be so desecrated. They read fairy tales together. Mr. Burroughs had disapproved of fairy tales. They blew soap-bubbles out on the lawn and let them float away over the garden and the orchard like fairy balloons. They had glorious afternoon teas under the beech tree. They made ice cream themselves. Jims even slid down the bannisters when he wanted to. And he could try out a slang word or two occasionally without anybody dying of horror. Miss Avery did not seem to mind it a bit.

At first Miss Avery always wore dark sombre dresses. But one day Jims found her in a pretty gown of pale primrose silk. It was very old and old-fashioned, but Jims did not know that. He capered round her in delight.

"You like me better in this?" she asked, wistfully.

"I like you just as well, no matter what you wear," said Jims, "but that dress is awfully pretty."

"Would you like me to wear bright colours, Jims?"

"You bet I would," said Jims emphatically.

After that she always wore them—pink and primrose and blue and white; and she let Jims wreathe flowers in her splendid hair. He had quite a knack of it. She never wore any jewellery except, always, a little gold ring with a design of two clasped hands.

"A friend gave that to me long ago when we were boy and girl together at school," she told Jims once. "I never take it off, night or day. When I die it is to be buried with me."

"You mustn't die till I do," said Jims in dismay.

"Oh, Jims, if we could only *live* together nothing else would matter," she said hungrily. "Jims—Jims—I see so little of you really—and some day soon you'll be going to school—and I'll lose you."

"I've got to think of some way to prevent it," cried Jims. "I won't have it. I won't—I won't."

But his heart sank notwithstanding.

One day Jims slipped from the blue room, down the pine and across the lawn with a tear-stained face.

"Aunt Augusta is going to kill my gobbler," he

sobbed in Miss Avery's arms. "She says she isn't going to bother with him any longer—and he's getting old—and he's to be killed. And that gobbler is the only friend I have in the world except you. Oh, I can't *stand* it, Miss Avery."

Next day Aunt Augusta told him the gobbler had been sold and taken away. And Jims flew into a passion of tears and protest about it and was promptly incarcerated in the blue room. A few minutes later a sobbing boy plunged through the trees—and stopped abruptly. Miss Avery was reading under the beech and the Black Prince was snoozing on her knee—and a big, magnificent, bronze turkey was parading about on the lawn, twisting his huge fan of a tail this way and that.

"*My* gobbler!" cried Jims.

"Yes. Martha went to your uncle's house and bought him. Oh, she didn't betray you. She told Nancy Jane she wanted a gobbler and, having seen one over there, thought perhaps she could get him. See, here's your pet, Jims, and here he shall live till he dies of old age. And I have something else for you—Edward and Martha went across the river yesterday to the Murray Kennels and got it for you."

"Not a dog?" exclaimed Jims.

"Yes—a dear little bull pup. He shall be your very own, Jims, and I only stipulate that you reconcile the Black Prince to him."

It was something of a task but Jims succeeded. Then followed a month of perfect happiness. At least three afternoons a week they contrived to be together. It was all too good to be true, Jims felt. Something would happen soon to spoil it. Just *suppose* Aunt Augusta grew tender-hearted and ceased to punish! Or suppose she suddenly discovered that he was growing too big to be shut up! Jims began to stint himself in eating lest he grew too fast. And then Aunt Augusta worried about his loss of appetite and suggested to Uncle Walter that he should be sent to the country till the hot weather was over. Jims didn't want to go to the country now because his heart was elsewhere. He must eat again, if he grew like a weed. It was all very harassing.

Uncle Walter looked at him keenly.

"It seems to me you're looking pretty fit, Jims. Do you want to go to the country?"

"No, please."

"Are you happy, Jims?"

"Sometimes."

"A boy should be happy all the time, Jims."

"If I had a mother and someone to play with I would be."

"I have tried to be a mother to you, Jims," said Aunt Augusta, in an offended tone. Then she addressed Uncle Walter. "A younger woman would probably understand him better. And I feel that the care of this big place is too much for me. I would prefer to go to my own old home. If you had married long ago, as you should, Walter, James would have had a mother and some cousins to play with. I have always been of this opinion."

Uncle Walter frowned and got up.

"Just because one woman played you false is no good reason for spoiling your life," went on Aunt Augusta severely. "I have kept silence all these years but now I am going to speak—and speak plainly. You should marry, Walter. You are young enough yet and you owe it to your name."

"Listen, Augusta," said Uncle Walter sternly. "I loved a woman once. I believed she loved me. She sent me back my ring one day and with it a message saying she had ceased to care for me and bidding me never to try to look upon her face again. Well, I have obeyed her, that is all."

"There was something strange about all that, Walter. The life she has since led proves that. So you should not let it embitter you against all women."

"I haven't. It's nonsense to say I'm a woman-hater, Augusta. But that experience has robbed me of the power to care for another woman."

"Well, this isn't a proper conversation for a child to hear," said Aunt Augusta, recollecting herself. "Jims, go out."

Jims would have given one of his ears to stay and listen with the other. But he went obediently.

And then, the very next day, the dreaded something happened.

It was the first of August and very, very hot. Jims was late coming to dinner and Aunt Augusta reproved him and Jims, deliberately, and with malice aforethought, told her he thought she was a nasty old woman. He had never been saucy to Aunt Augusta before. But it was three days since he had seen Miss Avery and the Black Prince and Nip and he was desperate. Aunt Augusta crimsoned with anger and doomed Jims to an afternoon in the blue room for impertinence.

"And I shall tell your uncle when he comes home," she added.

That rankled, for Jims didn't want Uncle Walter to think him impertinent. But he forgot all his worries as he scampered through the Garden of Spices to the beech tree. And there Jims stopped as if he had been shot. Prone on the grass under the beech tree, white and cold and still, lay his Miss Avery—dead, stone dead!

At least Jims thought she was dead. He flew into the house like a mad thing, shrieking for Martha. Nobody answered. Jims recollected, with a rush of sickening dread, that Miss Avery had told him Martha and Edward were going away that day to visit a sister. He rushed blindly across the lawn again, through the little side gate he had never passed before and down the street home. Uncle Walter was just opening the door of his car.

"Uncle Walter—come—come," sobbed Jims, clutching frantically at his hand. "Miss Avery's dead—dead—oh, come quick."

"*Who* is dead?"

"Miss Avery—Miss Avery Garland. She's lying on the grass over there in her garden. And I love her so—and I'll die, too—oh, Uncle Walter, *come*."

Uncle Walter looked as if he wanted to ask some questions, but he said nothing. With a strange face he hurried after Jims. Miss Avery was still lying there. As Uncle Walter bent over her he saw the broad red scar and started back with an exclamation.

"She is dead?" gasped Jims.

"No," said Uncle Walter, bending down again—"no, she has only fainted, Jims—overcome by the heat, I suppose. I want help. Go and call somebody."

"There's no one home here to-day," said Jims, in a spasm of joy so great that it shook him like a leaf.

"Then go home and telephone over to Mr. Loring's. Tell them I want the nurse who is there to come here for a few minutes."

Jims did his errand. Uncle Walter and the nurse carried Miss Avery into the house and then Jims went back to the blue room. He was so unhappy he didn't care where he went. He wished something *would* jump at him out of the bed and put an end to him. Everything was discovered now and he would never see Miss Avery again. Jims lay very still on the window seat. He did not even cry. He had come to one of the griefs that lie too deep for tears.

"I think I must have been put under a curse at birth," thought poor Jims.

Over at the stone house Miss Avery was lying on the couch in her room. The nurse had gone away and Dr. Walter was sitting looking at her. He leaned forward and pulled away the hand with which she was hiding the scar on her face. He looked first at the little gold ring on the hand and then at the scar.

"Don't," she said piteously.

"Avery—why did you do it?—*why* did you do it?"

"Oh, you know—you must know now, Walter."

"Avery, did you break my heart and spoil my life—and your own—simply because your face was scarred?"

"I couldn't bear to have you see me hideous," she moaned. "You had been so proud of my beauty. I—I—thought you couldn't love me any more—I couldn't bear the thought of looking in your eyes and seeing aversion there."

Walter Grant leaned forward.

"Look in my eyes, Avery. Do you see any aversion?"

Avery forced herself to look. What she saw covered her face with a hot blush.

"Did you think my love such a poor and superficial thing, Avery," he said sternly, "that it must vanish because a blemish came on your fairness? Do you think *that* would change me? Was your own love for me so slight?"

"No—no," she sobbed. "I have loved you every

269

moment of my life, Walter. Oh, don't look at me so sternly."

"If you had even told me," he said. "You said I was never to try to look on your face again—and they told me you had gone away. You sent me back my ring."

"I kept the old one," she interrupted, holding out her hand, "the first one you ever gave me—do you remember, Walter? When we were boy and girl."

"You robbed me of all that made life worthwhile, Avery. Do you wonder that I've been a bitter man?"

"I was wrong—I was wrong," she sobbed. "I should have believed in you. But don't you think I've paid, too? Forgive me, Walter—it's too late to atone—but forgive me."

"*Is* it too late?" he asked gravely.

She pointed to the scar.

"Could you endure seeing this opposite to you every day at your table?" she asked bitterly.

"Yes—if I could see your sweet eyes and your beloved smile with it, Avery," he answered passionately. "Oh, Avery, it was *you* I loved—not your outward favour. Oh, how foolish you were—foolish and morbid! You always put too high a value on beauty, Avery. If I had dreamed of the true state of the case—if I had known you were here all these years—why I heard a rumour long ago that you had married, Avery—but if I had known I would have come to you and *made* you be—sensible."

She gave a little laugh at his lame conclusion. That was so like the old Walter. Then her eyes filled with tears as he took her in his arms.

The door of the blue room opened. Jims did not look up. It was Aunt Augusta, of course—and she had heard the whole story.

"Jims, boy."

Jims lifted his miserable eyes. It was Uncle Walter—but a different Uncle Walter—an Uncle Walter with laughing eyes and a strange radiance of youth about him.

"Poor, lonely little fellow," said Uncle Walter unexpectedly. "Jims, would you like Miss Avery to come *here*—and live with us always—and be your real aunt?"

"Great snakes!" said Jims, transformed in a second. "Is there any chance of *that*?"

"There is a certainty, thanks to you," said Uncle Walter. "You can go over to see her for a little while. Don't talk her to death—she's weak yet—and attend to that menagerie of yours over there—she's worrying because the bull dog and gobbler weren't fed—and Jims—"

But Jims had swung down through the pine and was tearing across the Garden of Spices.

GIOVANNI BOCCACCIO

Day 5, novel IV of The Decameron

—Ricciardo Manardi is found by Messer Lizio da Valbona with his daughter, whom he marries, and remains at peace with her father.—

In silence Elisa received the praise bestowed on her story by her fair companions; and then the queen called for a story from Filostrato, who with a laugh began on this wise:—Chidden have I been so often and by so many of you for the sore burden, which I laid upon you, of discourse harsh and meet for tears, that, as some compensation for such annoy, I deem myself bound to tell you somewhat that may cause you to laugh a little: wherefore my story, which will be of the briefest, shall be of a love, the course whereof, save for sighs and a brief passage of fear mingled with shame, ran smooth to a happy consummation.

Know then, noble ladies, that 'tis no long time since there dwelt in Romagna a right worthy and courteous knight, Messer Lizio da Valbona by name, who was already verging upon old age, when, as it happened, there was born to him of his wife, Madonna Giacomina, a daughter, who, as she grew up, became the fairest and most debonair of all the girls of those parts, and, for that she was the only daughter left to them, was most dearly loved and cherished by her father and mother, who guarded her with most jealous care, thinking to arrange some great match for her. Now there was frequently in

273

Messer Lizio's house, and much in his company, a fine, lusty young man, one Ricciardo de' Manardi da Brettinoro, whom Messer Lizio and his wife would as little have thought of mistrusting as if he had been their own son: who, now and again taking note of the damsel, that she was very fair and graceful, and in bearing and behaviour most commendable, and of marriageable age, fell vehemently in love with her, which love he was very careful to conceal. The damsel detected it, however, and in like manner plunged headlong into love with him, to Ricciardo's no small satisfaction. Again and again he was on the point of speaking to her, but refrained for fear; at length, however, he summoned up his courage, and seizing his opportunity, thus addressed her:— "Caterina, I implore thee, suffer me not to die for love of thee." Whereto the damsel forthwith responded:— "Nay, God grant that it be not rather that I die for love of thee." Greatly exhilarated and encouraged, Ricciardo made answer:—" 'Twill never be by default of mine that thou lackest aught that may pleasure thee; but it rests with thee to find the means to save thy life and mine." Then said the damsel:—"Thou seest, Ricciardo, how closely watched I am, insomuch that I see not how 'twere possible for thee to come to me; but if thou seest aught that I may do without dishonour, speak the word, and I will do it." Ricciardo was silent a while, pondering many matters: then, of a sudden, he said:—"Sweet my Caterina, there is but one way that I can see, to wit, that thou shouldst sleep either on or where thou mightst have access to the terrace by thy father's garden, where, so I but knew that thou wouldst be there at night, I would without fail contrive to meet thee, albeit 'tis very high." "As for my sleeping there," replied Caterina, "I doubt not that it may be managed, if thou art sure that

274

thou canst join me." Ricciardo answered in the affirmative. Whereupon they exchanged a furtive kiss, and parted.

On the morrow, it being now towards the close of May, the damsel began complaining to her mother that by reason of the excessive heat she had not been able to get any sleep during the night. "Daughter," said the lady, "what heat was there? Nay, there was no heat at all." "Had you said, 'to my thinking,' mother," rejoined Caterina, "you would perhaps have said sooth; but you should bethink you how much more heat girls have in them than ladies that are advanced in years." "True, my daughter," returned the lady, "but I cannot order that it shall be hot and cold, as thou perchance wouldst like; we must take the weather as we find it, and as the seasons provide it: perchance to-night it will be cooler, and thou wilt sleep better." "God grant it be so," said Caterina, "but 'tis not wonted for the nights to grow cooler as the summer comes on." "What then," said the lady, "wouldst thou have me do?" "With your leave and my father's," answered Caterina, "I should like to have a little bed made up on the terrace by his room and over his garden, where, hearing the nightingales sing, and being in a much cooler place, I should sleep much better than in your room." Whereupon:—"Daughter, be of good cheer," said the mother; "I will speak to thy father, and we will do as he shall decide." So the lady told Messer Lizio what had passed between her and the damsel; but he, being old and perhaps for that reason a little morose, said:—"What nightingale is this, to whose chant she would fain sleep? I will see to it that the cicadas shall yet lull her to sleep." Which speech, coming to Caterina's ears, gave her such offence, that for anger, rather than by reason of the heat, she not only slept not herself that night, but suffered not her mother to sleep, keeping up a perpetual complaint of the great heat. Wherefore her mother hied her in the morning to Messer Lizio, and said to him:—"Sir, you hold your daughter none too dear; what difference can it make to you that she lie on the terrace? She has tossed about all night long by reason of the heat; and besides, can you wonder that she, girl that she is, loves to hear the nightingale sing? Young folk naturally affect their likes." Whereto Messer Lizio made answer:—"Go, make her a bed there to your liking, and set a curtain round it, and let her sleep there, and hear the nightingale sing to her heart's content." Which the damsel no sooner learned, than she had a bed made there with intent to sleep there that same night; wherefore she watched until she saw Ricciardo, whom by a concerted sign she gave to understand what he was to do. Messer Lizio, as soon as he had heard the damsel go to bed, locked a door that led from his room to the terrace, and went to sleep himself. When all was quiet, Ricciardo with the help of a ladder got upon a wall, and standing thereon laid hold of certain toothings of another wall, and not without great exertion and risk, had he fallen, clambered up on to the terrace, where the damsel received him quietly with the heartiest of cheer. Many a kiss they exchanged; and then got them to bed, where well-nigh all night long they had solace and joyance of one another, and made the nightingale sing not a few times. But, brief being the night and great their pleasure, towards dawn, albeit they wist it not, they fell asleep, Caterina's right arm encircling Ricciardo's neck, while with her left hand she held him by that part of his person which your modesty, my ladies, is most averse to name in the company of men. So, peacefully they slept, and were still asleep when day broke and Messer Lizio rose; and calling to mind that his daughter slept on the terrace, softly opened the door, saying to himself:—Let me see what sort of night's rest the nightingale has afforded our Caterina? And having entered, he gently raised the curtain that screened the bed, and saw Ricciardo asleep with her and in her embrace as described, both being quite naked and uncovered; and having taken note of Ricciardo, he went away, and hied him to his lady's room, and called her, saying:—"Up, up, wife, come and see; for thy daughter has fancied the nightingale to such purpose that she has caught him, and holds him in her hand." "How can this be?" said the lady. "Come quickly, and thou shalt see," replied Messer Lizio. So the lady huddled on her clothes, and silently followed Messer Lizio, and when they were come to the bed, and had raised the curtain, Madonna Giacomina saw plainly enough how her daughter had caught, and did hold the nightingale, whose song she had so longed to hear. Whereat the lady, deeming that Ricciardo had played her a cruel trick, would have cried out and upbraided him; but Messer Lizio said to her:—"Wife, as thou valuest my love, say not a word; for in good sooth, seeing that she has caught him, he shall be hers. Ricciardo is a gentleman and wealthy; an alliance with him cannot but be to our advantage: if he would part from me on good terms, he must first marry her, so that the nightingale shall prove to have been put in his own cage and not in that of another." Whereby the lady was reassured, seeing that her husband took the affair so quietly, and that her daughter had had a good night, and was rested, and had caught the nightingale. So she kept silence; nor had they long to wait before Ricciardo awoke; and, seeing that 'twas broad day, deemed that 'twas as much as his life was worth, and aroused Caterina, saying:—"Alas! my soul, what shall we do, now that day has come and surprised me here?" Which question Messer Lizio answered by coming forward, and saying:—"We shall do well." At sight of him Ricciardo felt as if his heart were torn out of his body, and sate up in the bed, and said:—"My lord, I cry you mercy for God's sake. I wot that my disloyalty and delinquency have merited death; wherefore deal with me even as it may seem best to you: however, I pray you, if so it may be, to spare my life, that I die not." "Ricciardo," replied Messer Lizio, "the love I bore thee, and the faith I reposed in thee, merited a better return; but still, as so it is, and youth has seduced thee into such a transgression, redeem thy life, and preserve my honour, by making Caterina thy lawful spouse, that thine, as she has been for this past night, she may remain for the rest of her life. In this way thou mayst secure my peace and thy safety; otherwise commend thy soul to God." Pending this colloquy, Caterina let go the nightingale, and having covered herself, began with many a tear to implore her father to forgive Ricciardo, and Ricciardo to do as Messer Lizio required, that thereby they might securely count upon a long continuance of such nights of delight. But there needed not much supplication; for, what with remorse for the wrong done, and the wish to make amends, and the fear of death, and the desire to escape it, and above all ardent love, and the craving to possess the beloved one, Ricciardo lost no time in making frank avowal of his readiness to do as Messer Lizio would have him. Wherefore Messer Lizio, having borrowed a ring from Madonna Giacomina, Ricciardo did there and then in their presence wed Caterina. Which done, Messer Lizio and the lady took their leave, saying:—"Now rest ye a while; for so perchance 'twere better for you than if ye rose." And so they left the young folks, who forthwith embraced, and not having travelled more than six miles during the night, went two miles further before they rose, and so concluded their first day. When they were risen, Ricciardo and Messer Lizio discussed the matter with more formality; and some days afterwards Ricciardo, as was meet, married the damsel anew in presence of their friends and kinsfolk, and brought her home with great pomp, and celebrated his nuptials with due dignity and splendour. And so for many a year thereafter he lived with her in peace and happiness, and snared the nightingales day and night to his heart's content.

FLORA ANNIE STEEL

The Bogey-Beast

There was once a woman who was very, very cheerful, though she had little to make her so; for she was old, and poor, and lonely. She lived in a little bit of a cottage and earned a scant living by running errands for her neighbours, getting a bite here, a sup there, as reward for her services. So she made shift to get on, and always looked as spry and cheery as if she had not a want in the world.

Now one summer evening, as she was trotting, full of smiles as ever, along the high road to her hovel, what should she see but a big black pot lying in the ditch!

"Goodness me!" she cried, "that would be just the very thing for me if I only had something to put in it! But I haven't! Now who could have left it in the ditch?"

And she looked about her expecting the owner would not be far off; but she could see nobody.

"Maybe there is a hole in it," she went on, "and that's why it has been cast away. But it would do fine to put a flower in for my window; so I'll just take it home with me."

And with that she lifted the lid and looked inside. "Mercy me!" she cried, fair amazed. "If it isn't full of gold pieces. Here's luck!"

And so it was, brim-full of great gold coins. Well, at first she simply stood stock-still, wondering if she was standing on her head or her heels. Then she began saying:

"Lawks! But I do feel rich. I feel awful rich!"

After she had said this many times, she began to wonder how she was to get her treasure home. It was too heavy for her to carry, and she could see no better way than to tie the end of her shawl to it and drag it behind her like a go-cart.

"It will soon be dark," she said to herself as she trotted along. "So much the better! The neighbours will not see what I'm bringing home, and I shall have all the night to myself, and be able to think what I'll do! Mayhap I'll buy a grand house and just sit by the fire with a cup o' tea and do no work at all like a queen. Or maybe I'll bury it at the garden foot and just keep a bit in the old china teapot on the chimney-piece. Or maybe—Goody! Goody! I feel that grand I don't know myself."

By this time she was a bit tired of dragging such a heavy weight, and, stopping to rest a while, turned to look at her treasure.

And lo! it wasn't a pot of gold at all! It was nothing but a lump of silver.

She stared at it, and rubbed her eyes, and stared at it again.

"Well! I never!" she said at last. "And me thinking it was a pot of gold! I must have been dreaming. But this is luck! Silver is far less trouble—easier to mind, and not so easy stolen. Them gold pieces would have been the death o' me, and with this great lump of silver—"

So she went off again planning what she would do, and feeling as rich as rich, until becoming a bit tired again she stopped to rest and gave a look round to see if her treasure was safe; and she saw nothing but a great lump of iron!

"Well! I never!" says she again. "And I mistaking it

for silver! I must have been dreaming. But this is luck! It's real convenient. I can get penny pieces for old iron, and penny pieces are a deal handier for me than your gold and silver. Why! I should never have slept a wink for fear of being robbed. But a penny piece comes in useful, and I shall sell that iron for a lot and be real rich—rolling rich."

So on she trotted full of plans as to how she would spend her penny pieces, till once more she stopped to rest and looked round to see her treasure was safe. And this time she saw nothing but a big stone.

"Well! I never!" she cried, full of smiles. "And to think I mistook it for iron. I must have been dreaming. But here's luck indeed, and me wanting a stone terrible bad to stick open the gate. Eh my! but it's a change for the better! It's a fine thing to have good luck."

So, all in a hurry to see how the stone would keep the gate open, she trotted off down the hill till she came to her own cottage. She unlatched the gate and then turned to unfasten her shawl from the stone which lay on the path behind her. Aye! It was a stone sure enough. There was plenty light to see it lying there, douce and peaceable as a stone should.

So she bent over it to unfasten the shawl end, when—"Oh my!" All of a sudden it gave a jump, a squeal, and in one moment was as big as a haystack. Then it let down four great lanky legs and threw out two long ears, nourished a great long tail and romped off, kicking and squealing and whinnying and laughing like a naughty, mischievous boy!

The old woman stared after it till it was fairly out of sight, then she burst out laughing too.

"Well!" she chuckled, "I am in luck! Quite the lucki-est body hereabouts. Fancy my seeing the Bogey-Beast

283

all to myself; and making myself so free with it too! My goodness! I do feel that uplifted—that *GRAND*!"—

So she went into her cottage and spent the evening chuckling over her good luck.

The Bamboo Cutter and the Moon Child

Long, long ago, there lived an old bamboo wood-cutter. He was very poor and sad also, for no child had Heaven sent to cheer his old age, and in his heart there was no hope of rest from work till he died and was laid in the quiet grave. Every morning he went forth into the woods and hills wherever the bamboo reared its lithe green plumes against the sky. When he had made his choice, he would cut down these feathers of the forest, and splitting them lengthwise, or cutting them into joints, would carry the bamboo wood home and make it into various articles for the household, and he and his old wife gained a small livelihood by selling them.

One morning as usual he had gone out to his work, and having found a nice clump of bamboos, had set to work to cut some of them down. Suddenly the green grove of bamboos was flooded with a bright soft light, as if the full moon had risen over the spot. Looking round in astonishment, he saw that the brilliance was streaming from one bamboo. The old man, full of wonder, dropped his axe and went towards the light. On nearer approach he saw that this soft splendour came from a hollow in the green bamboo stem, and still more wonderful to behold, in the midst of the brilliance stood a tiny human being, only three inches in height, and exquisitely beautiful in appearance.

"You must be sent to be my child, for I find you here among the bamboos where lies my daily work," said the old man, and taking the little creature in his hand he took it home to his wife to bring up. The tiny girl was so exceedingly beautiful and so small, that the old woman put her into a basket to safeguard her from the least possibility of being hurt in any way.

The old couple were now very happy, for it had been a lifelong regret that they had no children of their own, and with joy they now expended all the love of their old age on the little child who had come to them in so marvellous a manner.

From this time on, the old man often found gold in the notches of the bamboos when he hewed them down and cut them up; not only gold, but precious stones also, so that by degrees he became rich. He built himself a fine house, and was no longer known as the poor bamboo woodcutter, but as a wealthy man.

Three months passed quickly away, and in that time the bamboo child had, wonderful to say, become a full-grown girl, so her foster-parents did up her hair and dressed her in beautiful kimonos. She was of such wondrous beauty that they placed her behind the screens like a princess, and allowed no one to see her, waiting upon her themselves. It seemed as if she were made of light, for the house was filled with a soft shining, so that even in the dark of night it was like daytime. Her presence seemed to have a benign influence on those there. Whenever the old man felt sad, he had only to look upon his foster-daughter and his sorrow vanished, and he became as happy as when he was a youth.

At last the day came for the naming of their new-found child, so the old couple called in a celebrated name-giver, and he gave her the name of Princess Moonlight, because her body gave forth so much soft bright light that she might have been a daughter of the Moon God.

For three days the festival was kept up with song and dance and music. All the friends and relations of the old couple were present, and great was their enjoyment of the festivities held to celebrate the naming of Princess Moonlight. Everyone who saw her declared that there never had been seen anyone so lovely; all the beauties throughout the length and breadth of the land would grow pale beside her, so they said. The fame of the Princess's loveliness spread far and wide, and many were the suitors who desired to win her hand, or even so much as to see her.

Suitors from far and near posted themselves outside the house, and made little holes in the fence, in the hope of catching a glimpse of the Princess as she went from one room to the other along the veranda. They stayed there day and night, sacrificing even their sleep for a chance of seeing her, but all in vain. Then they approached the house, and tried to speak to the old man and his wife or some of the servants, but not even this was granted them.

Still, in spite of all this disappointment they stayed on day after day, and night after night, and counted it as nothing, so great was their desire to see the Princess.

At last, however, most of the men, seeing how hopeless their quest was, lost heart and hope both, and returned to their homes. All except five Knights, whose ardour and determination, instead of waning, seemed to wax greater with obstacles. These five men even went without their meals, and took snatches of whatever they could get brought to them, so that they might always stand outside the dwelling. They stood there in all weathers, in sunshine and in rain.

Sometimes they wrote letters to the Princess, but no answer was vouchsafed to them. Then when letters failed to draw any reply, they wrote poems to her telling her of the hopeless love which kept them from sleep, from food, from rest, and even from their homes. Still Princes Moonlight gave no sign of having received their verses.

In this hopeless state the winter passed. The snow and frost and the cold winds gradually gave place to the gentle warmth of spring. Then the summer came, and the sun burned white and scorching in the heavens above and on the earth beneath, and still these faithful Knights kept watch and waited. At the end of these long months they called out to the old bamboo-cutter and entreated him to have some mercy upon them and to show them the Princess, but he answered only that as he was not her real father he could not insist on her obeying him against her wishes.

The five Knights on receiving this stern answer returned to their several homes, and pondered over the best means of touching the proud Princess's heart, even so much as to grant them a hearing. They took their rosaries in hand and knelt before their household shrines, and burned precious incense, praying to Buddha to give them their heart's desire. Thus several days passed, but even so they could not rest in their homes.

So again they set out for the bamboo-cutter's house. This time the old man came out to see them, and they asked him to let them know if it was the Princess's resolution never to see any man whatsoever, and they implored him to speak for them and to tell her the greatness of their love, and how long they had waited through the cold of winter and the heat of summer, sleepless and roofless through all weathers, without food and without rest, in the ardent hope of winning her, and they were willing to consider this long vigil as pleasure if she would but give them one chance of pleading their cause with her.

The old man lent a willing ear to their tale of love, for in his inmost heart he felt sorry for these faithful suitors and would have liked to see his lovely foster-daughter married to one of them. So he went in to Princess Moonlight and said reverently:

"Although you have always seemed to me to be a heavenly being, yet I have had the trouble of bringing you up as my own child and you have been glad of the protection of my roof. Will you refuse to do as I wish?"

Then Princess Moonlight replied that there was nothing she would not do for him, that she honoured and loved him as her own father, and that as for herself she could not remember the time before she came to earth.

The old man listened with great joy as she spoke these dutiful words. Then he told her how anxious he was to see her safely and happily married before he died.

"I am an old man, over seventy years of age, and my end may come any time now. It is necessary and right that you should see these five suitors and choose one of them."

"Oh, why," said the Princess in distress, "must I do this? I have no wish to marry now."

"I found you," answered the old man, "many years ago, when you were a little creature three inches high, in the midst of a great white light. The light streamed from the bamboo in which you were hid and led me to you. So I have always thought that you were more than mortal woman. While I am alive it is right for you to remain as you are if you wish to do so, but someday I shall cease to be and who will take care of you then? Therefore I pray you to meet these five brave men one at a time and make up your mind to marry one of them!"

Then the Princess answered that she felt sure that she was not as beautiful as perhaps report made her out to be, and that even if she consented to marry any one of them, not really knowing her before, his heart might change afterwards. So as she did not feel sure of them, even though her father told her they were worthy Knights, she did not feel it wise to see them.

"All you say is very reasonable," said the old man, "but what kind of men will you consent to see? I do not call these five men who have waited on you for months, light-hearted. They have stood outside this house through the winter and the summer, often denying themselves food and sleep so that they may win you. What more can you demand?"

Then Princess Moonlight said she must make further trial of their love before she would grant their request to interview her. The five warriors were to prove their love by each bringing her from distant countries something that she desired to possess.

That same evening the suitors arrived and began to play their flutes in turn, and to sing their self-composed songs telling of their great and tireless love. The bamboo-cutter went out to them and offered them his sympathy for all they had endured and all the patience they had shown in their desire to win his foster-daughter. Then he gave them her message, that she would consent to marry whosoever was successful in bringing her what she wanted. This was to test them.

The five all accepted the trial, and thought it an

excellent plan, for it would prevent jealousy between them.

Princess Moonlight then sent word to the First Knight that she requested him to bring her the stone bowl which had belonged to Buddha in India.

The Second Knight was asked to go to the Mountain of Horai, said to be situated in the Eastern Sea, and to bring her a branch of the wonderful tree that grew on its summit. The roots of this tree were of silver, the trunk of gold, and the branches bore as fruit white jewels.

The Third Knight was told to go to China and search for the fire-rat and to bring her its skin.

The Fourth Knight was told to search for the dragon that carried on its head the stone radiating five colours and to bring the stone to her.

The Fifth Knight was to find the swallow which carried a shell in its stomach and to bring the shell to her.

The old man thought these very hard tasks and hesitated to carry the messages, but the Princess would make no other conditions. So her commands were issued word for word to the five men who, when they heard what was required of them, were all disheartened and disgusted at what seemed to them the impossibility of the tasks given them and returned to their own homes in despair.

But after a time, when they thought of the Princess, the love in their hearts revived for her, and they resolved to make an attempt to get what she desired of them.

The First Knight sent word to the Princess that he was starting out that day on the quest of Buddha's bowl, and he hoped soon to bring it to her. But he had not the courage to go all the way to India, for in those days traveling was very difficult and full of danger, so he went to one of the temples in Kyoto and took a stone bowl from the altar there, paying the priest a large sum of money for it. He then wrapped it in a cloth of gold and, waiting quietly for three years, returned and carried it to the old man.

Princess Moonlight wondered that the Knight should have returned so soon. She took the bowl from its gold wrapping, expecting it to make the room full of light, but it did not shine at all, so she knew that it was a sham thing and not the true bowl of Buddha. She returned it at once and refused to see him. The Knight threw the bowl away and returned to his home in despair. He gave up now all hopes of ever winning the Princess.

The Second Knight told his parents that he needed change of air for his health, for he was ashamed to tell them that love for the Princess Moonlight was the real cause of his leaving them. He then left his home, at the same time sending word to the Princess that he was setting out for Mount Horai in the hope of getting her a branch of the gold and silver tree which she so much wished to have. He only allowed his servants to accompany him half-way, and then sent them back. He reached the seashore and embarked on a small ship, and after sailing away for three days he landed and employed several carpenters to build him a house contrived in such a way that no one could get access to it. He then shut himself up with six skilled jewellers, and endeavoured to make such a gold and silver branch as he thought would satisfy the Princess as having come from the wonderful tree growing on Mount Horai. Every one whom he had asked declared that Mount Horai belonged to the land of fable and not to fact.

When the branch was finished, he took his journey home and tried to make himself look as if he were wearied and worn out with travel. He put the jewelled branch into a lacquer box and carried it to the bamboo-cutter, begging him to present it to the Princess.

The old man was quite deceived by the travel-stained appearance of the Knight, and thought that he had only just returned from his long journey with the branch. So he tried to persuade the Princess to consent to see the man. But she remained silent and looked very sad. The old man began to take out the branch and praised it as a wonderful treasure to be found nowhere in the whole land. Then he spoke of the Knight, how handsome and how brave he was to have undertaken a journey to so remote a place as the Mount of Horai.

Princess Moonlight took the branch in her hand and looked at it carefully. She then told her foster-parent that she knew it was impossible for the man to have obtained a branch from the gold and silver tree growing on Mount Horai so quickly or so easily, and she was sorry to say she believed it artificial.

The old man then went out to the expectant Knight, who had now approached the house, and asked where he had found the branch. Then the man did not scruple to make up a long story.

"Two years ago I took a ship and started in search of Mount Horai. After going before the wind for some time I reached the far Eastern Sea. Then a great storm arose and I was tossed about for many days, losing all count of the points of the compass, and finally we were blown ashore on an unknown island. Here I found the place inhabited by demons who at one time threatened to kill and eat me. However, I managed to make friends with these horrible creatures, and they helped me and my sailors to repair the boat, and I set sail again. Our food gave out, and we suffered much from sickness on board. At last, on the five-hundredth day from the day of starting, I saw far off on the horizon what looked like the peak of a mountain. On nearer approach, this proved to be an island, in the centre of which rose a high mountain. I landed, and after wandering about for two or three days, I saw a shining being coming towards me on the beach, holding in his hands a golden bowl. I went up to him and asked him if I had, by good chance, found the island of Mount Horai, and he answered:"

"'Yes, this is Mount Horai!'"

"With much difficulty I climbed to the summit, here stood the golden tree growing with silver roots in the ground. The wonders of that strange land are many, and if I began to tell you about them I could never stop. In spite of my wish to stay there long, on breaking off the branch I hurried back. With utmost speed it has taken me four hundred days to get back, and, as you see, my clothes are still damp from exposure on the long sea voyage. I have not even waited to change my raiment, so anxious was I to bring the branch to the Princess quickly."

Just at this moment the six jewellers, who had been employed on the making of the branch, but not yet paid by the Knight, arrived at the house and sent in a petition to the Princess to be paid for their labour. They said that they had worked for over a thousand days making the branch of gold, with its silver twigs and its jewelled fruit, that was now presented to her by the Knight, but as yet they had received nothing in payment. So this Knight's deception was thus found out, and the Princess, glad of an escape from one more importunate suitor, was only too pleased to send back the branch. She called in the workmen and had them paid liberally, and they went away happy. But on the way home they were overtaken by the disappointed man, who beat them till they were nearly dead, for letting out the secret, and they barely escaped with their lives. The Knight then returned home, raging in his heart; and in despair of ever winning the Princess gave up society and retired to a solitary life among the mountains.

Now the Third Knight had a friend in China, so he wrote to him to get the skin of the fire-rat. The virtue of any part of this animal was that no fire could harm it. He promised his friend any amount of money he liked to ask if only he could get him the desired article. As soon as the news came that the ship on which his friend had sailed home had come into port, he rode seven days on horseback to meet him. He handed his friend a large sum of money, and received the fire-rat's skin. When he reached home he put it carefully in a box and sent it in to the Princess while he waited outside for her answer.

The bamboo-cutter took the box from the Knight and, as usual, carried it in to her and tried to coax her to see the Knight at once, but Princess Moonlight refused, saying that she must first put the skin to test by putting it into the fire. If it were the real thing it would not burn. So she took off the crape wrapper and opened the box, and then threw the skin into the fire. The skin crackled and burnt up at once, and the Princess knew that this man also had not fulfilled his word. So the Third Knight failed also.

Now the Fourth Knight was no more enterprising than the rest. Instead of starting out on the quest of the dragon bearing on its head the five-colour-radiating jewel, he called all his servants together and gave them the order to seek for it far and wide in Japan and in

China, and he strictly forbade any of them to return till they had found it.

His numerous retainers and servants started out in different directions, with no intention, however, of obeying what they considered an impossible order. They simply took a holiday, went to pleasant country places together, and grumbled at their master's unreasonableness.

The Knight meanwhile, thinking that his retainers could not fail to find the jewel, repaired to his house, and fitted it up beautifully for the reception of the Princess, he felt so sure of winning her.

One year passed away in weary waiting, and still his men did not return with the dragon-jewel. The Knight became desperate. He could wait no longer, so taking with him only two men he hired a ship and commanded the captain to go in search of the dragon; the captain and the sailors refused to undertake what they said was an absurd search, but the Knight compelled them at last to put out to sea.

When they had been but a few days out they encountered a great storm which lasted so long that, by the time its fury abated, the Knight had determined to give up the hunt of the dragon. They were at last blown on shore, for navigation was primitive in those days. Worn out with his travels and anxiety, the fourth suitor gave himself up to rest. He had caught a very heavy cold, and had to go to bed with a swollen face.

The governor of the place, hearing of his plight, sent messengers with a letter inviting him to his house. While he was there thinking over all his troubles, his love for the Princess turned to anger, and he blamed her for all the hardships he had undergone. He thought that it was quite probable she had wished to kill him so that she might be rid of him, and in order to carry out her wish had sent him upon his impossible quest.

At this point all the servants he had sent out to find the jewel came to see him, and were surprised to find praise instead of displeasure awaiting them. Their master told them that he was heartily sick of adventure, and said that he never intended to go near the Princess's house again in the future.

Like all the rest, the Fifth Knight failed in his quest—he could not find the swallow's shell.

By this time the fame of Princess Moonlight's beauty had reached the ears of the Emperor, and he sent one of the Court ladies to see if she were really as lovely as report said; if so he would summon her to the Palace and make her one of the ladies-in-waiting.

When the Court lady arrived, in spite of her father's entreaties, Princess Moonlight refused to see her. The Imperial messenger insisted, saying it was the Emperor's order. Then Princess Moonlight told the old man that if she was forced to go to the Palace in obedience to the Emperor's order, she would vanish from the earth.

When the Emperor was told of her persistence in refusing to obey his summons, and that if pressed to obey she would disappear altogether from sight, he determined to go and see her. So he planned to go on a hunting excursion in the neighbourhood of the bamboo-cutter's house, and see the Princess himself. He sent word to the old man of his intention, and he received consent to the scheme. The next day the Emperor set out with his retinue, which he soon managed to outride. He found the bamboo-cutter's house and dismounted. He then entered the house and went straight to where the Princess was sitting with her attendant maidens.

Never had he seen anyone so wonderfully beautiful, and he could not but look at her, for she was more lovely than any human being as she shone in her own soft radiance. When Princess Moonlight became aware that a stranger was looking at her she tried to escape from the room, but the Emperor caught her and begged her to listen to what he had to say. Her only answer was to hide her face in her sleeves.

The Emperor fell deeply in love with her, and begged her to come to the Court, where he would give her a position of honour and everything she could wish for. He was about to send for one of the Imperial palanquins to take her back with him at once, saying that her grace and beauty should adorn a Court, and not be hidden in a bamboo-cutter's cottage.

But the Princess stopped him. She said that if she were forced to go to the Palace she would turn at once into a shadow, and even as she spoke she began to lose her form. Her figure faded from his sight while he looked.

The Emperor then promised to leave her free if only she would resume her former shape, which she did.

It was now time for him to return, for his retinue would be wondering what had happened to their Royal master when they missed him for so long. So he bade her good-by, and left the house with a sad heart. Princess Moonlight was for him the most beautiful woman in the world; all others were dark beside her, and he thought of her night and day. His Majesty now spent much of his time in writing poems, telling her of his love and devotion, and sent them to her, and though she refused to see him again she answered with many verses of her own composing, which told him gently and kindly that she could never marry anyone on this earth. These little songs always gave him pleasure.

At this time her foster-parents noticed that night after night the Princess would sit on her balcony and gaze for hours at the moon, in a spirit of the deepest dejection, ending always in a burst of tears. One night the old man found her thus weeping as if her heart were broken, and he besought her to tell him the reason of her sorrow.

With many tears she told him that he had guessed rightly when he supposed her not to belong to this world—that she had in truth come from the moon, and that her time on earth would soon be over. On the fifteenth day of that very month of August her friends from the moon would come to fetch her, and she would have to return. Her parents were both there, but having spent a lifetime on the earth she had forgotten them, and also the moon-world to which she belonged. It made her weep, she said, to think of leaving her kind foster-parents, and the home where she had been happy for so long.

When her attendants heard this they were very sad, and could not eat or drink for sadness at the thought that the Princess was so soon to leave them.

The Emperor, as soon as the news was carried to him, sent messengers to the house to find out if the report were true or not.

The old bamboo-cutter went out to meet the Imperial messengers. The last few days of sorrow had told upon the old man; he had aged greatly, and looked much more than his seventy years. Weeping bitterly, he told them that the report was only too true, but he intended, however, to make prisoners of the envoys from the moon, and to do all he could to prevent the Princess from being carried back.

The men returned and told His Majesty all that had passed. On the fifteenth day of that month the Emperor sent a guard of two thousand warriors to watch the house. One thousand stationed themselves on the roof, another thousand kept watch round all the entrances of the house. All were well trained archers, with bows and arrows. The bamboo-cutter and his wife hid Princess Moonlight in an inner room.

The old man gave orders that no one was to sleep that night, all in the house were to keep a strict watch, and be ready to protect the Princess. With these precautions, and the help of the Emperor's men-at-arms, he hoped to withstand the moon-messengers, but the Princess told him that all these measures to keep her would be useless, and that when her people came for her nothing whatever could prevent them from carrying out their purpose. Even the Emperor's men would be powerless. Then she added with tears that she was very, very sorry to leave him and his wife, whom she had learned to love as her parents, that if she could do as she liked she would stay with them in their old age, and try to make some return for all the love and kindness they had showered upon her during all her earthly life.

The night wore on. The yellow harvest moon rose high in the heavens, flooding the world asleep with her golden light. Silence reigned over the pine and the bamboo forests, and on the roof where the thousand men-at-arms waited.

Then the night grew grey towards the dawn and all hoped that the danger was over—that Princess Moonlight would not have to leave them after all. Then suddenly the watchers saw a cloud form round the moon—and while they looked this cloud began to roll earthwards. Nearer and nearer it came, and every one saw with dismay that its course lay towards the house.

In a short time the sky was entirely obscured, till at last the cloud lay over the dwelling only ten feet off the ground. In the midst of the cloud there stood a flying chariot, and in the chariot a band of luminous beings. One amongst them who looked like a king and appeared to be the chief stepped out of the chariot, and, poised in air, called to the old man to come out.

"The time has come," he said, "for Princess Moonlight to return to the moon from whence she came. She committed a grave fault, and as a punishment was sent to live down here for a time. We know what good care you have taken of the Princess, and we have rewarded you for this and have sent you wealth and prosperity. We put the gold in the bamboos for you to find."

"I have brought up this Princess for twenty years and never once has she done a wrong thing, therefore the lady you are seeking cannot be this one," said the old man. "I pray you to look elsewhere."

Then the messenger called aloud, saying:

"Princess Moonlight, come out from this lowly dwelling. Rest not here another moment."

At these words the screens of the Princess's room slid open of their own accord, revealing the Princess shining in her own radiance, bright and wonderful and full of beauty.

The messenger led her forth and placed her in the chariot. She looked back, and saw with pity the deep sorrow of the old man. She spoke to him many comforting words, and told him that it was not her will to leave him and that he must always think of her when looking at the moon.

The bamboo-cutter implored to be allowed to accompany her, but this was not allowed. The Princess took off her embroidered outer garment and gave it to him as a keepsake.

One of the moon beings in the chariot held a wonderful coat of wings, another had a phial full of the Elixir of Life which was given the Princess to drink. She swallowed a little and was about to give the rest to the old man, but she was prevented from doing so.

The robe of wings was about to be put upon her shoulders, but she said:

"Wait a little. I must not forget my good friend the Emperor. I must write him once more to say good-by while still in this human form."

In spite of the impatience of the messengers and charioteers she kept them waiting while she wrote. She placed the phial of the Elixir of Life with the letter, and, giving them to the old man, she asked him to deliver them to the Emperor.

Then the chariot began to roll heavenwards towards the moon, and as they all gazed with tearful eyes at the receding Princess, the dawn broke, and in the rosy light of day the moon-chariot and all in it were lost amongst the fleecy clouds that were now wafted across the sky on the wings of the morning wind.

Princess Moonlight's letter was carried to the Palace. His Majesty was afraid to touch the Elixir of Life, so he sent it with the letter to the top of the most sacred mountain in the land. Mount Fuji, and there the Royal emissaries burnt it on the summit at sunrise. So to this day people say there is smoke to be seen rising from the top of Mount Fuji to the clouds.

Leo Tolstoy

The Three Questions

It once occurred to a certain king, that if he always knew the right time to begin everything; if he knew who were the right people to listen to, and whom to avoid; and, above all, if he always knew what was the most important thing to do, he would never fail in anything he might undertake.

And this thought having occurred to him, he had it proclaimed throughout his kingdom that he would give a great reward to anyone who would teach him what was the right time for every action, and who were the most necessary people, and how he might know what was the most important thing to do.

And learned men came to the King, but they all answered his questions differently.

In reply to the first question, some said that to know the right time for every action, one must draw up in advance, a table of days, months and years, and must live strictly according to it. Only thus, said they, could everything be done at its proper time. Others declared that it was impossible to decide beforehand the right time for every action; but that, not letting oneself be absorbed in idle pastimes, one should always attend to all that was going on, and then do what was most needful. Others, again, said that however attentive the King might be to what was going on, it was impossible for one man to decide correctly the right time for every action, but that he should have a Council of wise men, who would help him to fix the proper time for everything.

But then again others said there were some things which could not wait to be laid before a Council, but about which one had at once to decide whether to undertake them or not. But in order to decide that, one must know beforehand what was going to happen. It is only magicians who know that; and, therefore, in order to know the right time for every action, one must consult magicians.

Equally various were the answers to the second question. Some said, the people the King most needed were his councillors; others, the priests; others, the doctors; while some said the warriors were the most necessary.

To the third question, as to what was the most important occupation: some replied that the most important thing in the world was science. Others said it was skill in warfare; and others, again, that it was religious worship.

All the answers being different, the King agreed with none of them, and gave the reward to none. But still wishing to find the right answers to his questions, he decided to consult a hermit, widely renowned for his wisdom.

The hermit lived in a wood which he never quitted, and he received none but common folk. So the King put on simple clothes, and before reaching the hermit's cell dismounted from his horse, and, leaving his bodyguard behind, went on alone.

When the King approached, the hermit was digging the ground in front of his hut. Seeing the King, he greeted him and went on digging. The hermit was frail and weak, and each time he stuck his spade into the ground and turned a little earth, he breathed heavily.

The King went up to him and said: "I have come to you, wise hermit, to ask you to answer three questions: How can I learn to do the right thing at the right time? Who are the people I most need, and to whom should I, therefore, pay more attention than to the rest? And, what affairs are the most important, and need my first attention?"

The hermit listened to the King, but answered nothing. He just spat on his hand and recommenced digging.

"You are tired," said the King, "let me take the spade and work awhile for you."

"Thanks!" said the hermit, and, giving the spade to the King, he sat down on the ground.

When he had dug two beds, the King stopped and repeated his questions. The hermit again gave no answer, but rose, stretched out his hand for the spade, and said:

"Now rest awhile—and let me work a bit."

But the King did not give him the spade, and continued to dig. One hour passed, and another. The sun began to sink behind the trees, and the King at last stuck the spade into the ground, and said:

"I came to you, wise man, for an answer to my questions. If you can give me none, tell me so, and I will return home."

"Here comes someone running," said the hermit, "let us see who it is."

The King turned round, and saw a bearded man come running out of the wood. The man held his hands pressed against his stomach, and blood was flowing from under them. When he reached the King, he fell fainting on the ground moaning feebly. The King and the hermit unfastened the man's clothing. There was a

large wound in his stomach. The King washed it as best
he could, and bandaged it with his handkerchief and
with a towel the hermit had. But the blood would not
stop flowing, and the King again and again removed the
bandage soaked with warm blood, and washed and re-
bandaged the wound. When at last the blood ceased
flowing, the man revived and asked for something to
drink. The King brought fresh water and gave it to him.
Meanwhile the sun had set, and it had become cool. So
the King, with the hermit's help, carried the wounded
man into the hut and laid him on the bed. Lying on the
bed the man closed his eyes and was quiet; but the King
was so tired with his walk and with the work he had
done, that he crouched down on the threshold, and also
fell asleep—so soundly that he slept all through the
short summer night. When he awoke in the morning, it
was long before he could remember where he was, or
who was the strange bearded man lying on the bed and
gazing intently at him with shining eyes.

"Forgive me!" said the bearded man in a weak voice,
when he saw that the King was awake and was looking
at him.

"I do not know you, and have nothing to forgive you
for," said the King.

"You do not know me, but I know you. I am that
enemy of yours who swore to revenge himself on you,
because you executed his brother and seized his property. I knew you had gone alone to see the hermit, and
I resolved to kill you on your way back. But the day
passed and you did not return. So I came out from my
ambush to find you, and I came upon your bodyguard,
and they recognized me, and wounded me. I escaped
from them, but should have bled to death had you
not dressed my wound. I wished to kill you, and you

have saved my life. Now, if I live, and if you wish it, I
will serve you as your most faithful slave, and will bid
my sons do the same. Forgive me!"

The King was very glad to have made peace with his
enemy so easily, and to have gained him for a friend,
and he not only forgave him, but said he would send
his servants and his own physician to attend him, and
promised to restore his property.

Having taken leave of the wounded man, the King
went out into the porch and looked around for the
hermit. Before going away he wished once more to beg
an answer to the questions he had put. The hermit was
outside, on his knees, sowing seeds in the beds that had
been dug the day before.

The King approached him, and said:

"For the last time, I pray you to answer my questions,
wise man."

"You have already been answered!" said the hermit
still crouching on his thin legs, and looking up at the
King, who stood before him.

"How answered? What do you mean?" asked the
King.

"Do you not see," replied the hermit. "If you had not
pitied my weakness yesterday, and had not dug those
beds for me, but had gone your way, that man would
have attacked you, and you would have repented of not
having stayed with me. So the most important time was
when you were digging the beds; and I was the most
important man; and to do me good was your most
important business. Afterwards when that man ran to
us, the most important time was when you were attending to him, for if you had not bound up his wounds he
would have died without having made peace with you.
So he was the most important man, and what you did

for him was your most important business. Remember then: there is only one time that is important—Now! It is the most important time because it is the only time when we have any power. The most necessary man is he with whom you are, for no man knows whether he will ever have dealings with anyone else: and the most important affair is, to do him good, because for that purpose alone was man sent into this life!

MACMILLAN COLLECTOR'S LIBRARY

Own the world's great works of literature in one beautiful collectible library

Designed and curated to appeal to book lovers everywhere, Macmillan Collector's Library editions are small enough to travel with you and striking enough to take pride of place on your bookshelf. These much-loved literary classics also make the perfect gift.

Beautifully produced with gilt edges, a ribbon marker, bespoke illustrated cover and real cloth binding, every Macmillan Collector's Library hardback adheres to the same high production values.

Discover something new or cherish your favourite stories with this elegant collection.

Macmillan Collector's Library: own, collect, and treasure

Discover the full range at
macmillancollectorslibrary.com

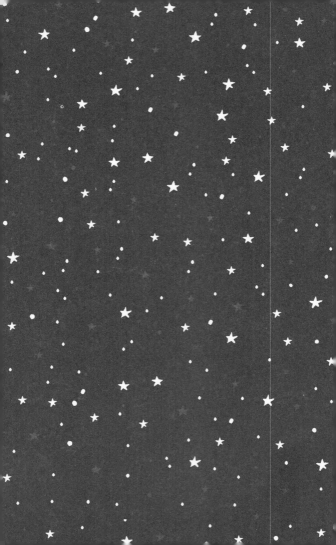